STAYING CONNECTED WHILE LETTING GO

The Paradox of Alzheimer's Caregiving

STAYING CONNECTED WHILE LETTING GO

The Paradox of Alzheimer's Caregiving

Sandy Braff and Mary Rose Olenik
Foreword by Arnold A. Lazarus, Ph.D., ABPP

M. Evans and Company, Inc.
New York

M. Evans and Company, Inc.
216 East 49th Street
New York, NY 10017

Library of Congress Cataloguing-in-Publication Data

Braff, Sandy.
Staying connected while letting go : the paradox of alzheimer's caregiving / by Sandy Braff and Mary Rose Olenik
p. cm.
ISBN 1-59077-012-9
1. Alzheimer's disease. 2. Caregivers. 3. Self-care, Health. I. Olenik, Mary Rose. II. Title.
RC523. B725 2002
616.8'31—dc21 200202731

Typesetting and design by Evan Johnston

Printed in the United States of America

9 8 7 6 5 4 3 2 1

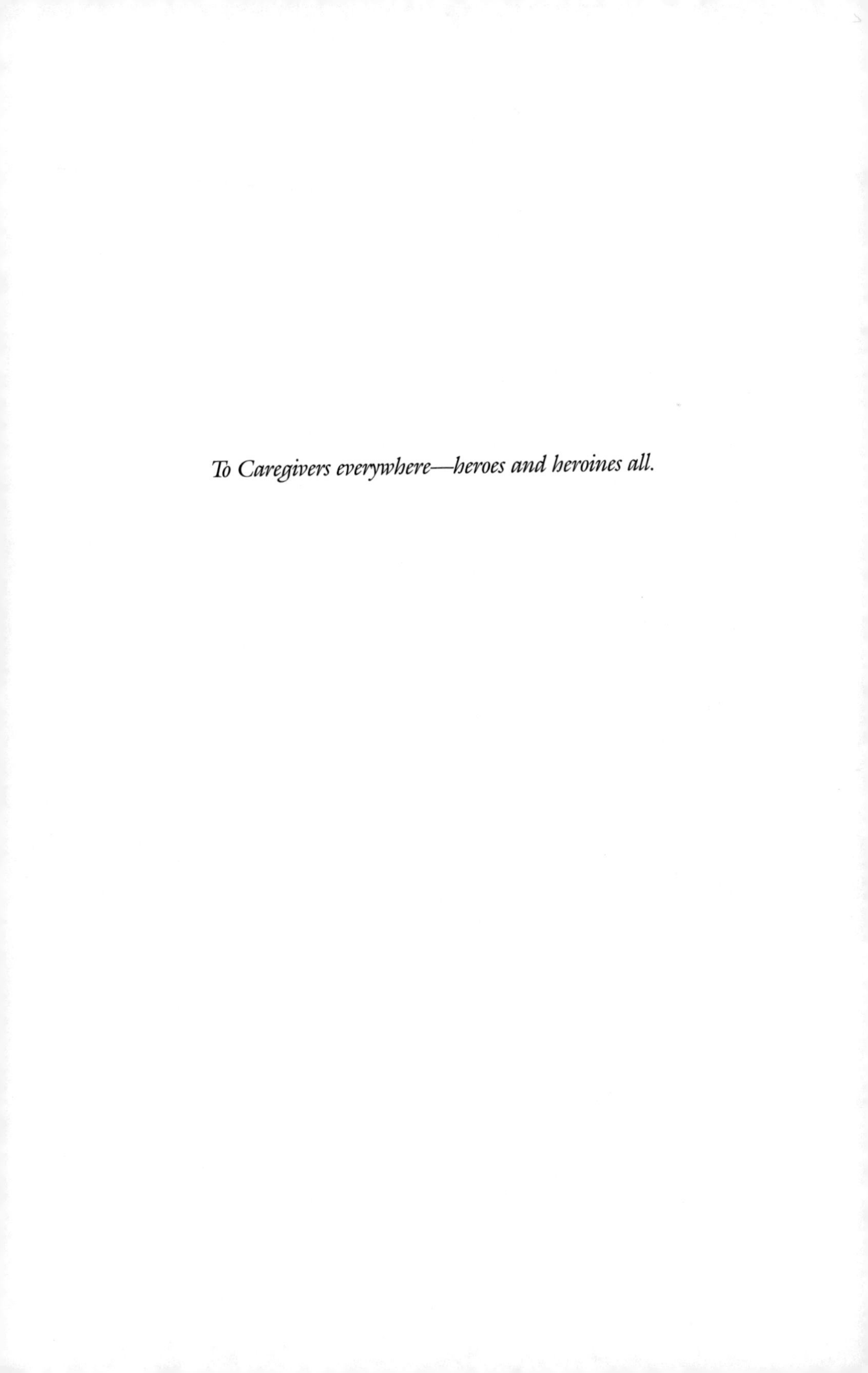

To Caregivers everywhere—heroes and heroines all.

CONTENTS

Foreword *xi*
Preface *xv*
Acknowledgments *xvi*
Introduction *1*

Part One: The Beginning Stage

Chapter 1. First Encounters **7**

Chapter 2. If Only I Could Be Wrong: Tentative Diagnosis **11**
Beginning Stage Behaviors • The Importance of Seeking a Diagnosis

Chapter 3. What Now? Reactions to the Diagnosis **21**
Disclosing the Diagnosis to the Patient • Disclosing the Diagnosis to Others • Legal and Financial Preparation

Chapter 4. Reaching In and Reaching Out: Adaptation **31**
Adaptation to Role Changes • Coping and Resilience

Chapter 5. Rallying the Troops: Family Reactions **39**

Chapter 6. The Shell Without the Pearl: Transcending Loss **45**
Loss of Mutuality • Loss of Personality • Loss of Communication • Loss of Physical Intimacy • Loss of Partnership • Loss of Sense of Belonging: Isolation • Discovering the Paradox of Caregiving

Part Two: The Middle Stage

Chapter 7. Coming to Terms 71

The Importance of Acquiring Coping Skills • Managing Your Attitudes and Thoughts • Middle-Stage Behaviors • Your Role in the Accomodating to the Middle Stage

Chapter 8. Confronting the Demons: Your Emotional Reactions to the Middle Stage 79

Denial • Resentment • Guilt • Fear • Frustration

Chapter 9. Tears of Laughter: The Importance of Humor 111

The Power of Laughter

Chapter 10. The Mars and Venus of Adapting to Change: Gender Differences 115

Chapter 11. The Lonely Bed: Adapting to Profound Loss of Intimacy 125

Understanding Sexual Behavior in Alzheimer's • Extramarital Companionship

Chapter 12. Harvesting Your Communal Garden: Preventing Burnout 135

• Taking Time out for Yourself • Day Care • In-home Care • Going It Alone

Chapter 13. I Think I Can, I Think I Can, I Know I Can: Resiliency 149

Coming to Terms with the Challenges of Alzheimer's

Part Three: The Late Middle Stage

Chapter 14. The Long Good-bye 157

• Late-Middle-Stage Behaviors • Loss of Recognition by Spouse

Chapter 15. I'm Beat and I'm Scared: Caregiving Intensifies—Resource Options 163

Family Involvement • Alternatives to Placement • When Placement Becomes Necessary • The Angst of Placement • Transitioning to Life Alone

Chapter 16. When Alone Equals Lonely: Loneliness and Companionship 189

Part Four: The Final Stage and Beyond

Chapter 17. Nearing the Journey's End: Final Stages of Alzheimer's 199

Final Stage Behaviors

Chapter 18. The Relief of Planning Ahead: Advanced Directives 207

Allowing for a Natural Death

Chapter 19. Another Paradox: Anticipatory Grief and Mourning 213

Chapter 20. At Peace, My Love: Death of a Spouse 217

Chapter 21. Cleaning out the Closets: The Process of Closure 227

Chapter 22. Honoring Your Tomorrows: Reentry Post Caregiving 231

Getting Started • Successfully Coming Full Circle • And You Shall Triumph

Bibliography 245
About the Authors 247
Index 249

Day by day blossoms alter and fall;
Year by year people transform and change
—Han-Shan

FOREWORD

Staying Connected While Letting Go: The Paradox of Alzheimer's Caregiving, brings to life the challenges and triumphs of courageous individuals who care for their loved ones who are afflicted with Alzheimer's disease. The authors shine an insightful, emotionally moving, and lyrical spotlight on a topic that is often ignored, minimized, or met with denial. They clearly articulate how caregivers can function as "full human beings" when so much of their energy is tied up in a relentless and inevitably losing battle with an unyielding enemy. Alzheimer's inescapably progresses from the initial stages of dementia through deeper and deeper levels of dysfunction across cognitive and behavioral domains. The authors have masterfully described how even the tragedy of Alzheimer's and the profoundly challenging tasks of caregiving can be transformed into a life-affirming process. The steps and strategies of this difficult process are illuminated in this outstanding book.

The wisdom and experience of the authors is subtly but distinctively infused throughout. The volume is structured by following caregivers and their loved ones through "First Encounters"—beginning stages—through "Coming to Terms" with the middle stages, and, finally,

"Nearing the Journey's End" and beyond, which describes the final stage. This clever "staging" of the major parts of the book parallels the course of the illness itself as told through the experiences, thoughts, and emotions of caregivers. The book describes the first subtle (and frequently denied) clues that a loved one is suffering from a significant cognitive and memory disturbance. Next, it addresses the tears, panic, and fear of a confirmed diagnosis; then the isolation and abandonment that caregivers experience in the lengthy middle stages; and finally the death of the spouse and the caregivers' reflections on their own transformation. Throughout the book other themes evolve—that losses can be acknowledged and transcended; that denial and anger can be constructively met with adaptive strategies and even humor; that family and friends can unite to support one another and utilize external and internal resources in their quest for achieving peace and tranquility rather than suffering the alternatives of isolation, despair, and fragmentation.

Ms. Braff's experience as a marriage family therapist enables her to assist caregivers and to facilitate her weekly Alzheimer's caregiver's support group, with which she has been involved for fifteen continuous years. She is able to help caregivers integrate how hope and cognitive reframing can offer productive compensatory strategies for caregivers. Ms. Olenik's six-year experience performing in-home evaluations of Alzheimer's caregivers in an important research project allows us to better understand the full impact of Alzheimer's disease on caregivers in their day-to-day struggles.

For caregivers and their families, this book offers unique insights into the workings of progressive dementia and its all-encompassing attack on what makes us truly human—our memories of the past, our awareness of the present, and our ability to plan for the future. But through this "veil of tears," the reader gradually learns adaptive strategies for dealing with his or her loved one's dementia and his or her own complex emotions from the earliest stages through mid and late disease states. The psychological approach includes the importance of early recognition and planning; developing a social support network; and adopting strategies for dealing with personal, legal, and ethical dilemmas. It is this rich vein of information and proven coping strategies that allows the reader to feel hopeful and inspired. Transforming fear into realistic planning and hope is not an easy prescription to write, but the authors have accomplished just that with kindness, compassion, reality testing, and proven adaptive strategies.

For **caregivers**, this book offers hope in the face of an unrelenting disease. For **relatives** and **friends**, it provides a deeper understanding of how they can help their loved ones in the depths of their despair. For the **health professionals**, who frequently see Alzheimer's patients for thirty minutes or less a week, the book offers an invaluable, realistic picture of what day-to-day life is like for Alzheimer's caregivers and their patients.

The authors have achieved an admirable and inspiring balance of realistic descriptions of the life and times of caregivers and a pathway by which survival and spiritual strength may be attained under difficult circumstances. Thus, for caregivers, their friends and family, and the medical and mental health communities, this book carries a compassionate but realistic and instructive message. It is a unique and inspiring message of hope and understanding. I recommend that all of the above groups who are touched by Alzheimer's carefully read and learn from this sensitively written and profoundly valuable book.

—Arnold A. Lazarus, Ph.D., ABPP
Distinguished Professor Emeritus of Psychology, Rutgers University

PREFACE

Some of the stories in this important book derive from experiences shared by participants of the University of California at San Diego Alzheimer's Caregiver Study, a program of research supported by the National Institutes of Health. In the fifteen years that I have had the privilege of leading this project, we have learned many things, some expected, others not. Yes, spouses who were providing care for a wife or husband with Alzheimer's disease did tend to have more health problems; some develop mild hypertension, others have alterations in their immune systems that might place them at risk to certain infectious diseases or cancers. There may be changes in blood factors that could increase the chance of heart disease or stroke.

But what we found more surprising was the remarkably good physical and emotional health of many caregivers. This resiliency has been less well investigated. And it is this theme that constitutes one of the fundamental messages that runs through this simply yet sensitively written book by Sandy Braff and Mary Rose Olenik.

I am delighted and very proud that Mary Rose, while working with our Study, dug into her creativity to begin integrating the many facets of caregiving into a human whole. Happily for all of us readers, she was able to weave her observations with those of Sandy Braff's long experience in caregiver support groups into a rich tapestry on spousal caregiving.

I am sure that the participants in the Alzheimer's Caregiver Study, who volunteered so generously of their time, will feel pleased that their stories and experiences contributed in some measure to a book that promises to provide information, comfort, and hope to all who face the challenges of Alzheimer's caregiving.

—Igor Grant, M.D.
Professor of Psychiatry and
Principal Investigator,
Alzheimer's Caregiver Study,
University of California,
San Diego

ACKNOWLEDGMENTS

The experience of writing a book about a recalcitrant illness and adverse emotions was, paradoxically, extraordinarily positive and life affirming for both of us. The process of our collaboration spawned a wonderful friendship between us, which was consistently buoyed by the extraordinary support, interest, and caring extended to us by our families, friends, and colleagues.

There are those who were particularly steadfast and to whom we are especially grateful:

Sandy's husband, Dave, who offered professional criticism and enduring support while retaining patience and humor, even upon being summarily evicted from our writing space.

Sandy's children, Dan and Lara Braff, for their pride and faith in this project and their excitement about the potential of this endeavor.

Mary Rose's daughter Andra Olenik, for her astute counsel in writing and publishing, and son Justin Olenik, for his encouragement and unwavering belief that our book would come to fruition.

Sandy's family in Johannesburg, South Africa: mother Doreen, sister Cynthia, niece Rahle, Uncle Len, and Mary for their belief in the worthiness of this book.

Paul Lapolla, our endearing, supportive sage, who has been inordinately attentive as our agent in fostering the success of our manuscript every step of the way.

Our publisher, George de Kay, and our editor, PJ Dempsey, for their flexibility, patience, and enthusiasm.

Dr. Trey Sutherland, Dr. Igor Grant, Dr. Kenneth Davis, Dr. Dilip Jeste, Dr. Aaron Beck, Stephen Winner, Lisa Gwyther MSW, Margee Frey, Joan Bosky, and caregivers Ann and Yvonne, who so generously took the time to read our manuscript and bowled us over with their positive comments and recommendations.

Our caregivers who shared their stories, which are the nucleus of our book, and whose wisdom and courage inspired us to write it.

INTRODUCTION

When we first met to talk about our experiences with caregivers and the possibility of writing a book together, we started sharing some of the marvelous stories that our caregivers had told us. We were deeply moved by the ordeals encountered by family caregivers and impressed by their ability to move beyond them. What evolved in our subsequent meetings was the recurring theme that, for caregivers, dealing with the practical and physical care of their patient was often more clearly understood and realizable than dealing with the profound emotional effects experienced by them in their cargiving role. We had consistently observed caregivers who were not taking care of their own emotional needs. The deleterious result was evidenced in their health, effectiveness, and stamina—a circumstance that often undermined their ability to adequately care for their patients.

We also realized that we had both been privy to a unique treasure chest of intimate, unequivocally honest and insightful stories told from the caregivers' perspectives about their journies through the vicissitudes of Alzheimer's disease caregiving. We concluded that these narrations should be the vehicle used in our book for discussing the emotional effects of caregiving throughout the progression of Alzheimer's disease, which robs the patient of the attributes and qualities that normally allow us to join and connect with each other in meaningful ways.

In these richly woven tales we have endeavored to set a unique and compassionate tone for caregivers, families, friends, physicians, and mental health professionals to facilitate their understanding of the day-to-day journey of navigating through the experience of Alzheimer's caregiving. The book opens a larger world for the perspectives of medical and mental health professionals as it vividly describes the 167+ hours in a caregiver's week, impossible to envision during a time-limited weekly or monthly office visit.

The stories, as told by actual caregivers, are narratives of grace, evolution, and transformation. Our caregivers' stories allow the reader into a sacred place that most people are not privy to: the deepest parts of their being in which their innermost thoughts are expressed. The depth of their emotions surfaces as they recount moments of crisis, of the absurd, of hopelessness and despair that are often counterbalanced by feelings of empowerment and triumph in coming to terms with this disease as well as with their role as caregiver. In *Staying Connected While Letting Go: The Paradox of Alzheimer's Caregiving*, we attempt to break down old assumptions, patterns, and expectations and offer alternative and imaginative ways of coping successfully. Our goal is to compassionately assist and encourage caregivers to change those thoughts and behaviors that inevitably sabotage not only the quality of care they give to their loved one, but also the way in which they attend to themselves. The book lends promise to the most discouraged caregiver as we ease the reader into a personal discovery of untapped potential that is rooted in his or her heretofore hidden strengths, coping skills, and ability to change. By using a cognitive therapy approach to facilitate this change, we teach our readers to alter their confusing and often defeatist concepts by coming to terms with and accepting without judgment their normal and often overwhelming negative emotions. The preeminent belief in this book is that it is necessary for caregivers to take care of their emotional selves, so that they have the internal strength to attend to their enormous task.

Sandy's stories were derived from her fifteen years of facilitating a weekly Alzheimer's caregiver support group for the San Diego Alzheimer's Association. We have chosen to use the stories from a core group of members of this particular group. Some of them have remained active in attendance for years and well beyond the death of their spouse. In the book you will also discover the importance of good support groups as you read their stories of camaraderie, compassion, and humor in that special setting.

As part of an Alzheimer's Caregiver Research Study at the University of California, San Diego, Mary Rose arranged for two-hour psychosocial interviews every six months with spousal caregivers who were the participants in the study. Over the six years of research, Mary Rose performed interviews with over 300 caregivers. Their stories were shared in those meetings that took place in the intimacy of their home, where Mary Rose could also observe the caregiver's environment and often the status of their Alzheimer's patient. Many of the vignettes you will read represent composites (to protect confidentiality) of stories that caregivers told Mary Rose during her interviews with them in the course of the UCSD Alzheimer's Caregiver Study, which was sponsored by the National Institutes of Health (NIH). I am grateful to Igor Grant, M.D., Study Principal Investigator, and to Thomas L. Patterson, Ph.D., Co-Investigator, for providing me with this opportunity to have access to caregivers and to hear their stories. I am especially thankful to the participants themselves, those caregivers who so generously opened their homes and heart to me and to the study.

A few of the caregivers in the book were in both Sandy's support group and Mary Rose's caregiver study. We have used artistic license and changed the names, places, and identifying features of all of the caregivers in order to preserve their rights to privacy and confidentiality.

In this book we honor caregivers everywhere. We hope that our deepest regard, admiration, and respect for all caregivers is manifested throughout its writing.

PART ONE
THE BEGINNING STAGE

CHAPTER 1

First Encounters

Paul

Feeling the weight of the day's events in every bone of his tall, slender body, Paul sank into his comfortable Stratolounger and switched on the table lamp. As he reached for the remote control so he could catch the late evening news, his eyes fixed on the photograph standing beside it. He picked it up instead and began to recall that wonderful day, only four years ago. He and Jane were in Maui, a vacation that the kids had given them to celebrate their fortieth wedding anniversary. Jane looked vibrant in her blue, flowered pareo and orchid lei. Paul, wearing his matching shirt, was standing next to her with his arm around her. Every day they had been snorkeling, and every night they danced into the wee hours. The last evening of the vacation, they stood on the veranda overlooking the ocean and repeated their wedding vows. Paul sighed deeply.

How things had changed! This morning, Jane had once again asked him where the bathroom was. He recalled how floored he had been the first time she seemed to be lost in their home of thirty-two years and thought at first that she had been joking. At lunch she accused Paul of having secret telephone conversations with her mother, who had been dead for years. That was a new one. He thought about how Jane, who used to love to cook, now frequently asked to go out to dinner. Pondering that recent turnaround, he recognized that Jane could not coordinate preparing even a simple dinner without his help.

Jane was asleep as Paul sat alone in the den, holding the photo close to his chest, painfully cognizant that their emotional bond—the essence of their partnership—was quickly slipping away.

Reluctantly, Paul admitted to himself that it was time to capitulate to the signs of an illness he had read about and feared to the depths of his soul. He knew he could no longer continue to ignore the probability that his beloved Jane had Alzheimer's disease. Placing the photograph back in its place on the table next to him, Paul rubbed his eyes, took a deep breath, and resolved that tomorrow would be a new day when a new journey would begin.

These "first encounters," which present themselves in various subtle and unusual behaviors, over time, initiate you into what is to become your role as a caregiver. Like Paul, a somewhat hazy and bewildering series of events may have you, your family, and friends shaking your heads and wondering, "what is going on here?" Not only are you thrown off balance, but you may also be frightened or even filled with disbelief and mixed emotions. Confronting these emotions causes perturbations that can disrupt your equilibrium and profoundly alter all significant relationships.

In our experience in working with the caregiving population, we have observed that each caregiver has a unique story to share about his or her encounter with Alzheimer's disease. These are stories of hope and courage in which caregivers like you, both heroes and heroines, demonstrate strength, endurance, and self-empowerment in order to clip the wings of and enfeeble the predatory emotional effects of Alzheimer's disease on your spouse, your family, and you. Those who succeed (and most of you do) learn how to confront the illness and to accept, rather than resist, the conflictual feelings that naturally arise, in order to restore your sense of competence and well-being. As time collaborates with you as a welcome friend and healer in this unpredictable and spasmodic venture, so does the fundamental support of friends and family.

CHAPTER 2

If Only I Could Be Wrong: Tentative Diagnosis

Angela

Since the support group's inception over nineteen years ago, Angela has been a regular participant. She freely shared her wisdom, gained through the experience of being a long-term caregiver. At one group meeting, where there were several new attendees, she recalled her first encounter with Alzheimer's disease.

> It has been about twenty years since Joe's first symptoms began. Looking back on our marriage, I would say that the first stages of this disease caused constant turmoil in our relationship. Yes, they really did. Those "early" years were sheer hell. We were always arguing. Then we would sit down together, discuss what had occurred, and I would feel we had worked this one out. The next day, guess what—we were at it again. Joe was also continually criticizing me, blaming me

for things that went wrong, real or imagined. Joe, who had always been easy to get along with, was acting irrationally. His judgment and reasoning were flawed. He was hypersensitive to criticism and even seemed somewhat paranoid. I could not figure out what had happened to him or to our marriage. In addition, much to my amazement, I later learned that he was complaining about my behavior to our daughters, who believed his interpretation of events.

During this time, I was experiencing stomach pains and other symptoms that, after many tests and consultations with various physicians and specialists, initially revealed no conclusive diagnosis. I thought I 5was going crazy. Only several years later did I see a doctor who believed that these symptoms were caused by what he referred to as a "masked depression." He prescribed an antidepressant for me at that time, which worked very well in reducing the symptoms.

In any case, out of sheer desperation and because my daughters were so insistent that their father was not functioning normally, I managed to persuade Joe to go to the doctor. Not an easy task. Once at the doctor's office, he had a thorough exam and the doctor told me he suspected that Joe was experiencing symptoms found in the early stages of Alzheimer's disease. As upsetting as this was for me to hear, I also experienced a sense of relief. At least now I had an idea about what was going on. At the same time, I thought, "This can't be so! This cannot be happening to Joe, to us, to our family."

Winston

Winston had found May's early symptoms unnerving. The more bewildered and confused May became, the more frustrated and impatient Winston became, resulting in an uncontrollable, impulsive, and regrettable act. He related with great pain in his voice:

My life with May had been so enjoyable before she became a victim of Alzheimer's disease. She was bright, energetic, articulate, and dignified. With me she was agreeable and calm, and always so understanding—in contrast to my impatience and quick temper. Over time she became increasingly moody, argumentative, and contrary. I found it infuriating. Her behavior had become a daily burden that perplexed and baffled me. My frustration and intolerance increased as she grew more cantankerous. We went to our family physician, who, after examining May, said he could find nothing wrong with her and suggested that she was just bored. I must admit, I was hoping for a more concrete answer. When I tried to involve May in more activities, she became worse, and noticeably inept. One day I lost it. I impulsively shoved May against the wall and yelled at her, telling her to shape up. Thank God, she was not injured, but I was horrified by what I had done. It was then that I knew I needed some answers, some help. I called my daughter in Chicago, who suggested that I take May to a neurologist. After performing many tests on her over the next few days, he finally diagnosed May as having "probable Alzheimer's." Finally, it all made sense. I began to see May as the victim of a terrible disease over which she had no control and I felt I had very little. I realized that I had to change the way I responded to May and I have. Slowly and painfully, I have had to come to terms with the reality that May is no longer the same person I fell in love with so many years ago, but we're still a team and we're going to stay that way.

In these stories we describe the subtle beginnings of what is finally diagnosed as "possible or probable Alzheimer's disease." Since the symptoms in the early stages of Alzheimer's disease are inconsistent and fairly unremarkable, it is common that it may be a few years from the time of their onset before a diagnosis is even sought. An occasional forgetful moment, a forgotten name, a misplaced article, even irrational irritable moments and nominal personality changes in the patient do not at first signify that something has gone awry.

The first encounters with Alzheimer's disease have far-reaching implications. Not only is a couple's relationship dramatically altered, but also, since our lives never exist in isolation, the effects can and often do impact many other relationships. Your personal world that includes children, other family members, friends, and community is also influenced by this formidable event. We compare the effects of these first encounters to the analogy of "the butterfly effect"—that is, the notion originating out of James Gleick's book, *Chaos Theory*, that a butterfly stirring the air today in Peking can ultimately transform storm systems the next month or the next year in New York. The subtle changes that are experienced at the beginning of Alzheimer's disease are pervasive, immutably transforming your world—beginning with your self-confidence and self-image and radiating virulently into marriage, relationships to family and friends, and society.

As we age, memory lapses are common and not necessarily a sign of possible Alzheimer's disease. We can all relate to the following statements:

"I simply cannot remember the author of the book I just finished reading!"

"What did I come into this room for?"

"Oh no, I did it again. Where did I park the car?"

BEGINNING STAGE BEHAVIORS

Most adults experience moments when they, too, draw a blank. In fact, these situations are universal. When, however, does forgetfulness become a clinically significant problem? What is the difference between simple forgetfulness, which becomes apparent as we age, and the memory loss evidenced in Alzheimer's disease? A more telling sign has to do with how new information is stored. Although we do slow down as we age, most elderly people can still store new information and also retrieve it later. However, a person who has Alzheimer's disease cannot learn new information or new tasks and does not have the ability to recall previously learned information. The cognitive characteristics of the beginning stage of Alzheimer's, which is usually diagnosed at around age sixty-five, are disturbances of one or more functions in language, motor skills, recognition, and identification of objects, and disturbances of executive functions such as planning, organizing, sequencing, or abstracting. You may notice changes in the personality of your loved one, perhaps loss of spontaneity, mood swings, anxiety, lack of initiative, or aggressive behavior.

The workings of the brain are marvelous and complicated. However, quite simply put, in the brain of the Alzheimer's patient, there is a progressive degeneration and loss of vast numbers of nerve cells in those portions of the brain's cortex that are associated with functions such as memory, learning, and judgment. The severity and nature of the patient's dementia at any given time are proportional to the number and location of cells that have been affected.

Because age-related memory problems at first glance are not clearly black and white and are fairly common in both older adults and in Alzheimer's patients, it's difficult to conclude when and if a diagnosis is warranted.

So what drives you to seek a diagnosis of your loved one? Sometimes the recognition of problem forgetfulness becomes very apparent at one moment in time, as it did to Hugh regarding his wife, Ellen.

Hugh

Although I recognized that my own memory was periodically unreliable, I noticed that Ellen was consistently forgetful, and I was getting a little worried about that. Then one afternoon when we were at the local shopping mall, I went in one direction and my bride went in the other, which is what we often did. We planned to meet at a particular restaurant at noon. Ellen showed up at the right time but with a single shoe under her arm. We both laughed that Ellen had absentmindedly taken

> the shoe from a store. I asked her, "Which store?" She had absolutely no idea, even after we had walked past every darn store in the shopping center, floor by floor, visiting every shoe store and department store in an attempt to return it. Don't even ask me what we finally did with the shoe.

Although at the time it seemed humorous, it was this glaring incident that exceeded the boundaries of ordinary forgetfulness and compelled Hugh to seek a diagnosis for Ellen.

Yvette

Yvette's experience with her husband, Richard, is a very different example ending with the same conclusion, the need for a definitive diagnosis. Richard's conduct was at times inappropriate and even appalling to Yvette. Sometimes he'd wear layers of clothing that were much too warm for temperate weather. However, it wasn't until his behavior began to spill out into the community, and it was glaringly obvious that Richard had lost his sense of societal boundaries, that Yvette sought a diagnosis.

> Richard began to wander out of the yard and take it upon himself to deliver the neighbors' mail or newspapers to them. He would take the mail out of their mailboxes and either knock on their front doors and hand it to them or would walk into their houses if the door was unlocked. At first, I didn't know that he was creating such havoc with the neighbors, until one very disgruntled neighbor called and complained to me about Richard. I was horrified, and apologized profusely. It seemed that no matter how many times I would remind him to refrain from handling the neighbors' mail, he would invariably forget and continue this inappropriate behavior. I began to feel that I was policing my husband and had to be constantly vigilant. I

bitterly resented this role. I was angry with the neighbors for their lack of compassion and with Richard for being out of control. I had attempted to explain that Richard was having memory problems, hoping they would be more empathic and patient with him, but what I really needed to do at that time was to realize myself that this was a real problem.

Sylvia

Phil's decline was, at first, more apparent with his job at an electronics manufacturer than it was at home. His supervisor called me and really caught me off guard. He explained that Phil's performance at work was slow and inefficient and his judgment and reasoning ability seemed increasingly impaired. Although this call was alarming, I began to make sense of Phil's avoidant behavior. He had begun to make excuses to stay home over the last month, and to avoid going to work. I had accepted this as he had seemed tired, and hence thought nothing of it.

At about the same time, I began to suspect that something was amiss when we received a couple of returned, inappropriately written checks and overdue notices. When I questioned Phil, he was quick to reassure me that he had everything under control. I always trusted him to pay the bills and chose to ignore the signs. However, after a few months, the errors increased and I decided to investigate. I was horrified when I discovered the chaotic state of our financial affairs.

This realization was difficult and complicated for Sylvia. Not only did she need to question and confront Phil about a task at which he had always been competent, but she also needed to come to terms with the painful reality that there was something wrong with his mind. With much trepidation, Sylvia approached Phil and told him what she had discovered. This difficult meeting for both Sylvia and Phil resulted in their scheduling an appointment with a neurologist after which Phil was ultimately diagnosed with "possible Alzheimer's" disease.

In one of our group discussions that centered around determining factors that ultimately led to a diagnosis, it was discovered that at times it is the affected spouse who will state that something is wrong, as was the case with Mannie's wife, Rachel.

Mannie

My wife, Rachel, feared that something was wrong with her brain. I had also noticed some changes in her memory and personality. Even though a tentative diagnosis would help us clarify whether or not Rachel had Alzheimer's, we were scared and reluctant to find out. She was also insistent that I not tell our children if the diagnosis was positive. Her mother had died of Alzheimer's, and she did not want to frighten them. At some point we realized that it was time to know if our worst fears were indeed a reality so that we could plan for our future accordingly. We went to the neurologist, who, after thorough examination, gave us the diagnosis of possible Alzheimer's disease. The churning inside me was terrible. We wanted to know and yet we didn't want to know. But there it was, and Rachel understood it and so did I. We went home, and for the next several days, we let it sink in and then began to get some legal work done and think about short- and long-term practical issues. I'm not sure we were ever closer or more appreciative of each other and what we had had all of these years together. Within the next few days, we broke the news to the children.

THE IMPORTANCE OF SEEKING A DIAGNOSIS

It is important to seek a diagnosis if warning signs are present. One of the reasons is that some forms of dementia can be treated. Never assume that, because your loved one is having these symptoms, he or she has Alzheimer's disease. If you must go through your primary care doctor for a referral, we encourage you to request a referral to a specialist such as a neurologist (M.D.) or a neuropsychologist (Ph.D.) for a detailed mental and physical examination. It's very important that someone who is familiar with the symptoms of early dementia related to Alzheimer's disease perform the evaluation and diagnosis of the patient. There are over one hundred illnesses that have symptoms similar to those found in the early stages of Alzheimer's disease. The right medication or other measures can help many of these dementia-like symptoms. For instance, some illnesses such as a brain tumor, Parkinson's disease, stroke, depression, or vitamin B–12 or folate deficiency may mimic the symptoms that appear as Dementia of the Alzheimer's Type (DAT). Your spouse should be given a thorough work-up that may include physical, neurological, and neuropsychological testing, as well as brain-imaging tests such as magnetic resonance imaging (MRI). The neuropsychological tests are detailed and reliable markers of cognitive function, including memory deficiency, while the MRI may show physical deterioration in the brain structure. Often, in the early stages, a definitive diagnosis cannot be made, so the best diagnosis at this time may be "possible" or "probable" Alzheimer's disease. A reliable diagnosis then calls for action on the part of the doctor as well as you, the caregiver. If there are memory problems, there are some medications that can aid in possibly slowing down the memory loss for a significant amount of time. If you live in an area where there is a university with an Alzheimer's research center, you might also want to consider enrolling your spouse as a participant or subject, where often the newest testing and drug trials are taking place. Many caregivers have told us that before the Alzheimer's diagnosis was made, they sought psychiatric help for their spouse, who may have been depressed or acting in an aberrant manner or because of the disruptive discord in their marital relationship. The psychiatrist who sees the patient will usually be able to discern that these problems could be related to the early symptoms of Alzheimer's disease and refer the patient for an appropriate evaluation.

Your role in the relationship may be difficult to sort out during this somewhat puzzling period, but you will discover that you learn and are able to adapt to changes, often without consciously realizing that you are doing so. Thank goodness for our ability to be resilient and to have the capacity to accommodate life's distressing experiences. Your personal journey toward transformation and metamorphosis begins as imperceptibly as the manifestation of Alzheimer's disease occurs in your loved one. By the journey's end, you will find that it is possible to grow stronger, develop new skills, and perhaps surprise yourself with how courageous, creative, and sturdy you really are.

CHAPTER 3

What Now? Reactions to the Diagnosis

Caregivers have many different reactions on hearing the diagnosis "probable Alzheimer's disease." If we recall Angela and Winston's stories, there was an initial sense of relief, because they finally knew what was causing their spouse's out-of-character behavior. That reaction is quite common and understandable. On the other hand, Bill's reaction was quite different on learning of his wife's diagnosis.

Bill

I took my wife, Hazel, to two different specialists. The second doctor we saw announced in front of Hazel that she probably had Alzheimer's disease. It was devastating to both of us to hear those words: "Alzheimer's disease." They seemed to burn in my mind. When we left the doctor's office, Hazel

> said to me, "I don't like those words, 'Alzheimer's disease.'" That was the only time she uttered that phrase out loud, and to this day, I have never used the label "Alzheimer's disease" in her presence. I believed it was up to me to deal with the reality of those words and protect my wife from ever having to confront them.

Most caregivers resonate with similar emotional experiences on hearing the diagnosis of probable Alzheimer's disease, sometimes disbelief, but more often relief and then apprehension. The positive outcome of the diagnosis is that it not only validates what many caregivers and their spouses have suspected, but it also moves them into action. The way that you, as a caregiver, proceed depends on many factors: your coping style, your attitude, your age and health, the status of the marital relationship, your past experience with a dementing illness, and most importantly, support from family and friends and available community resources. The more plentiful your resources are, the better you'll manage. Fortunately, these days, there are abundantly more resources being established in communities to provide the kind of assistance that you may need. Your local Alzheimer's Association is always a great place to start.

DISCLOSING THE DIAGNOSIS TO THE PATIENT

The question of whether or not to disclose the diagnosis to the patient is often discussed in the caregiver's support group. Ethically, the doctor is obliged to reveal the diagnosis to the patient. The question of whether or not the caregiver reinforces or reminds the patient of the diagnosis inevitably comes up. There is some controversy about how to handle this sensitive and crucial issue. Some professionals and caregivers believe that your patient ought to be told, which also conforms to a physician's ethical obligation to the patient, who at this stage of the disease is still functioning at a fairly high level. Since the patient is still capable, he or she is able to participate in legal and financial affairs and make choices about their lives. This could also allow for intimate conversations that might deepen connections with family and friends.

You will decide how to communicate about the disease with your loved one. Some of you will openly use the term "possible or probable Alzheimer's disease" in the presence of your ill spouse, while others, more cautious about your own as well as your spouse's ability to handle this diagnosis, will talk about "your memory problem" or the "problem with your brain." Whatever phrase you as a caregiver choose in explaining the symptomatic behavior in your spouse, we think it advisable that your choice defines the behavior as an illness, out of the patient's control, in order to protect the patient's self-esteem and integrity. In verbalizing this very important concept that the behavior is the illness, not the patient, you also begin to reinforce for yourself, especially as feelings of frustration, anger, or impatience begin to surface, that it is not your spouse but the illness.

Mamie

Very early in her husband's, Bud's, illness, Mamie was able to make a clear distinction, separating his disturbing behavior from his person, therefore effectively blaming the illness for his frustrating acts and preserving his dignity and self-respect.

During one of my visits to Mamie's home, Bud came storming into the room, oblivious of the fact that Mamie and I were conversing, and interrupted our interview. Frustrated and beside himself, he stammered, "I was in the garden and couldn't find the thing. You know, the thing that goes on the pipe that holds the other on the machine. I'm trying to put the water thing around the piece for the place on the wall. Damn it! I'm such a dunce!" He held his head in his hands, shaking it from side to side. Mamie had a very comforting and calming

> response. She said, "Daddy, don't get so mad at yourself. It's this crazy Alzheimer's that keeps you from remembering. Let's go outside together when Mary leaves and I'll help you. Now come sit down and I'll fix you some iced tea. You've been working so hard out there."

Bud immediately settled down and stopped berating himself. It was obvious in his eyes that he felt grateful to his wife, who had preserved his self-esteem. Although Mamie was saddened by Bud's incompetence, it was her ability to separate the disease from her husband and maintain control of her emotions that allowed her to communicate gently and lovingly, preventing these frequent situations from intensifying and diminishing Bud's self-worth.

The above example gives insight into a positive way of communicating with your spouse in the face of the anomalous and disturbing behaviors that are caused by Alzheimer's disease. Understandably, a lack of communication might also be due to your own fears and inability to face the reality of Alzheimer's disease at this time. However, it may be more negative and constrictive if there is no discussion between spouses about the disease itself, as the impact of the behaviors on the relationship are quite real.

Without a clear strategy of how and what to communicate with a spouse who has dementia, you may begin to feel powerless in the way you manage your patient and overwhelmed by your mixed emotions. You may continue to indict or become angry with your spouse instead of directing your anger at the real culprit, Alzheimer's disease. Since your spouse can no longer learn new skills, the onus is on you, the caregiver, to adapt and adjust to a new way of communicating. Successful interactions will depend not only on your flexibility, but also on your consistency and willingness to practice these new skills every day. We will discuss strategies throughout the book.

DISCLOSING THE DIAGNOSIS TO OTHERS

There are many different ways you will discover to talk to your spouse about the illness, and many different reasons why you may be reluctant to be candid about the illness with your children, other family members, and friends. We have observed that caregivers can be very creative in the way they choose to inform family or friends about their spouse's condition. There is no right or wrong way to do this. However, since there are real benefits in disclosure and open communication about the illness, you do need to find a way that feels comfortable for you.

In the following two examples, the first caregiver chose not to disclose any information about her husband's illness to anyone outside of the family. In the second example, the caregiver creatively informed his family and friends about his wife's diagnosis.

Jane

Jane, a quiet, unassuming woman from a small town in the Midwest, explained her reluctance to talk about her husband's illness.

> We lived in a small community in which we were very active. My husband, Mac, was a doctor, well known by everyone. I knew how he felt about people gossiping, and I decided, out of respect for him, that I would not say anything about his condition. I was aware that some people would raise an eyebrow at something he said or did, but simply chose to ignore their nonverbal behaviors. One day, he and a friend went golfing together. Shortly after Mac arrived home, I received a phone call from his friend's wife, Shirley, who told me that another golfing friend had brought her husband home, because my husband had simply left without him! Although I knew that he

was experiencing early signs of Alzheimer's disease, I said nothing to her.

Jane never did talk to her friends in Nebraska about Mac's Alzheimer's. She simply shrugged and said, *"I decided that they would eventually figure things out on their own, like Shirley probably did."*

Jane was resolute when she said that, out of respect for her husband, she would not talk about him, and even in the support group she attended, she spoke very little. As we learn along the way and as with many caregivers, her silence was based on her own denial. It was too painful for her to accept Mac's condition. She was also very stoic and did not want to lose control of herself emotionally. Jane wanted to be strong for her husband's sake and for the sake of their four adult children, who in turn wanted to abide by their mother's wishes.

This is an example of a caregiver who chose inordinate measures to avoid telling others about her husband's diagnosis. Yet, in not telling anyone, she could be jeopardizing her husband's safety. Also, because of her silence, she did not have the support of anyone who could have lightened her burden. As Mac's condition worsened, Jane made the decision to move to the West Coast, where they would be close to their son.

It seemed easier for her to admit to her husband's Alzheimer's in a new community of relative strangers. However, without a history and established friendships, she had very little support in her new community. It wasn't until, at her son's insistence, she joined a support group that she received adequate understanding and encouragement and felt a sense of belonging.

Tom

Tom and Joan were in their early sixties and very active, especially in doing volunteer work in their community. Tom's wife was in the early stage of Alzheimer's disease, and at the time of my first visit with him, the only person he had told about Joan's diagnosis was their daughter. On my subsequent visit, six months later, he described small but increasingly noticeable changes in his wife and said that he really had to learn to be more patient. They were volunteering together now and not separately. He said that in their annual Christmas letter, he had told his friends and relatives of the diagnosis of Alzheimer's disease. Tom described to me the sense of relief he had in no longer keeping this secret, and the wonderful, understanding, and supportive responses he and his wife had received from the recipients of the letter.

Many caregivers have asked how and when you ought to say something about your spouse's condition to other people. It is best to be open with family, friends, and even neighbors as soon as possible, for many reasons beyond the safety and needs of your patient. First, sharing this information decreases the isolation you may experience. Second, as in the case of Tom, you may feel an immense sense of relief, because it requires a lot of emotional energy to suppress all of these strong feelings. Finally, openly discussing the situation with family and friends tends to decrease the amount of confusion that already exists, and will also make space for people to ask questions or to be supportive and offer assistance. Ideally, this will encourage family and friends to find a role in your challenging plight that will be helpful and compassionate and will reduce your experience of being alone.

Too often, caregivers are reticent about asking for assistance for fear of rejection or out of pride or reluctance of becoming a burden. You might erroneously presume that you will not receive the help and understanding that you desperately need. However, the consequence of taking a risk and opening the door to communication is usually beneficial. It eliminates the ambiguity that you could experience in your relationships with friends and family. The durability of friendships becomes apparent. Those friends who accept the invitation and step through the door not only provide comfort by their presence, but also the assurance that the relationship is immutable and reliable. Just ask!

The early stages of Alzheimer's are an opportune time to take another risk by venturing outside of your known social circle to a support group or experienced mental health practitioner who understands precisely what caregivers in your situation experience. The relief of having a common language, of feeling understood, of communicating openly and frankly about the daily challenges presents the opportunity for both camaraderie and education that is beneficial to all caregivers.

On the lighter side, exchanging ideas in this forum often creates a joyful experience in which you can act silly, make jokes, and laugh at some of the absurdities that are part and parcel of this illness. This may sound contradictory and certainly irreverent, but we have observed many caregiver who, despite their tears in describing an upsetting occurrence, will burst out laughing at the foolishness or absurdity conveyed in the telling. A little levity goes a long way in normalizing a situation.

LEGAL AND FINANCIAL PREPARATION

It is vital in these early stages that you and your family communicate with your legal and financial advisors about preparing a Durable Power of Attorney for Health Care (DPAHC) and Durable Power of Attorney for Finances (DPAF) as well as a living will for your spouse and yourself if that has not yet been accomplished. State laws vary on what is necessary and may vary in the names of necessary documents, but for the most part they are fairly straightforward.

It is advantageous to get the signature of your spouse while he or she is competent to sign. Otherwise these legal matters can become more problematic and expensive, for example, if legal conservatorship must be obtained. While he or she is still able, it may also be necessary to have your spouse's help in locating assets. Clearly these are vital details that can impact the entire family.

The DPAHC allows another person to be appointed to make decisions about what types of medical care your spouse should receive if unconscious or unable to make decisions on his or her own. The DPAHC differs from a living will. The living will states the person's desire not to receive life-sustaining treatment if terminally ill or in an irreversible coma. The DPAF gives you power over all legal and financial matters. Durable Powers of Attorney are honored in all fifty states, although there may be some variation in the language. If you don't have a legal advisor—and we suggest an attorney whose expertise is in elder law—often the Alzheimer's Association in your area can give you recommendations.

CHAPTER 4

Reaching In and Reaching Out: Adaptation

During the initial phase of Alzheimer's disease, which can last for many years, caregivers like you have proved themselves capable of adapting to the aberrant behaviors and other changes in their loved one. However, initially, an enormous amount of energy might be spent protecting your relationship with your spouse: trying to keep it as it was and living in hope from day to day that things will be different tomorrow, for things to be as they were. Perhaps human nature is always trying to maintain a homeostasis or equilibrium—to retain balance in the midst of turmoil. Alzheimer's comes with an enormous cache of turmoil, which can lead to a gradual decline in the quality of your life and, in some caregivers, a static existence in which you become completely immersed in the mire of caregiving. You must become vigilant and realistic about knowing yourself and your limitations. Usually, in time, with the passing of day into night and night into day again, and as many tomorrows come and go, you find that you do habituate to each situation and all its inconsistencies and move forward.

We emphasize that, in order to facilitate adjusting to the task of caregiving, it is important that you, the caregiver, see yourself as a whole person, a complete individual in your own right, separate from your spouse. Who were you before marriage, before the onset of your spouse's disease? What interests, pleasures, and attributes defined you, independent of the marriage? Can you embrace those attributes and qualities that make you who you are and keep a healthy boundary between you and this confounding predicament in which you find yourself? Hopefully, as you read the stories in this book and discover how other caregivers have adjusted, you will tap into your exceptional and possibly dormant inner strength and discover that you can adapt and accommodate and still retain a sense of self—a self that also needs care, nurturing, and pleasurable activities.

Adaptation occurs differently for each person, due to the complex nature of relationships as well as individual coping styles and temperaments. Since the disease progresses through different stages as your loved one declines, you will discover that each stage seems to reach a plateau when your spouse "levels off" for a while, forcing you to adjust by modifying your behavior and accommodating new challenges. Alzheimer's disease is deceptive and guileful. It lures you into believing a status quo has been established. You begin to feel more or less content with your ability to cope, and out of the blue, a new deterioration or crisis appears, a new plateau is reached, and so begins another cycle of adjustment and reassessment. Living with this unstable state of affairs predicated on the whims of Alzheimer's is quite difficult, but despite the tribulations, ultimately, you will adapt and learn to cope.

ADAPTATION TO ROLE CHANGES

The following are three examples of adaptation to caregiving. In the first story, you will see that Yvette had a great deal of difficulty. The second example, Neil's, illustrates how the caregiver, although struggling at the outset, eventually realized that he had been seduced by the power of denial, and this realization evolved into a helpful tool in adjusting to his new role. Finally, in the third example, Tony gives a positive lesson in adapting throughout the various stages of the disease.

Yvette

> From the very beginning of Richard's illness, I struggled to understand what had happened to my husband of forty years. Rich had been a very capable man, on whom I had grown to depend almost completely. As he gradually became less functional due to his dementia, he was unable to carry out or complete even the simplest tasks, like paying the bills or picking up groceries. I often feel overwhelmed and even guilty. Reluctantly, I've been forced to take over the finances.
>
> After the doctor recommended that Rich stop driving, I went to the DMV to take Rich's name off the car and have his license revoked, and then gave the car to our son. As the law requires, our doctor also wrote a letter to the DMV, stating that Rich had been diagnosed with possible Alzheimer's. When Rich questioned me about the car and I told him what I had done, I realized it was the first time I'd made any major decision without consulting him. Then I told him we could buy him a new car if he felt he needed to drive, knowing in my own mind that that would never happen. I felt awful knowing that I was dishonest with him.
>
> I feel incompetent and insecure in making all of the decisions and taking on these new responsibilities. I'm constantly worried that I'm not doing the right thing, and I can't ask Rich for feedback. I feel terribly insecure and unsure of myself.

Yvette's lack of self-confidence and poor coping skills were debilitating. She complained bitterly to the group over and over again. The members patiently encouraged Yvette to take one day at a time so that she would not feel so overwhelmed. They continued to give her positive reinforcement for the accomplishments she had made, like taking over the finances and making a realistic decision about Richard continuing to drive the car. They also consistently and gently reinforced the notion that Richard would not get better, and consequently, Yvette would need to continue to summon her strength, but they would be there for her.

Perhaps the reason for her reluctance to make any changes was that Yvette, like most caregivers, was clinging to the hope that the disease would magically reverse itself and Rich would get better, not worse. This example of denial commonly occurs in the early stages of the illness, particularly when the patient continues to have periods of lucidity. When the "shades are up," you find yourself face-to-face with the same person you always knew and loved. Hope rises. Doubts about the accuracy of the diagnosis lure you into wishful thinking. Then suddenly the "shades go down," and once again you grieve and long for that person who has disappeared again. How ambiguous and tormenting!

In Yvette's mind, possibly, yielding to the role change would also mean she was surrendering to the illness. Combined with the negative messages she was sending to herself about her ability to cope with new and changing responsibilities, she remained in a rut of pessimism.

Neil

When I look back at the way I handled Denise in the early stages of her disease, I recall how reluctant I was to tell the neighbors anything about her. Every day she would go for walks alone in the neighborhood, which seemed to me to be pretty safe. It wasn't a matter of getting lost, but one day, she tripped and fell as she approached the house. Fortunately, I happened to be watching for her, and when I saw her fall, I rushed outside to help her. Denise was very shaken and confused, and I noticed immediately that she was unable to get up on her own. A neighbor ran out at about that same time and helped me get Denise back into the house. That incident finally shook me into reality. Immediately afterward, I began to tell all of our neighbors about her condition. I now realize that my silence had to do with my own fear and denial. I still didn't want to believe that Denise was afflicted with Alzheimer's disease. I thought that in holding out and keeping this from the neighbors, I didn't have to admit it to myself. Like it didn't have to be real yet. After she fell, I realized that I was jeopardizing Denise's safety. As I talk, I understand the power of denial and how it had me in its grip. When I began telling the neighbors, I had finally begun to acknowledge the disturbing truth about Denise's illness.

Tony

We can all take heart from Tony's story.

In the past, Sophie, upon awakening, would bring a cup of hot coffee up to Tony, as he was getting ready for work. Tony could remember fondly how Sophie had pampered him. Because of Sophie's illness, he was now compelled to adjust and create new routines. For months, it was Tony who now prepared their breakfast while Sophie awakened and dressed. In spite of this role-reversal, a comfortable morning ritual evolved. One morning, however, after calling his wife to breakfast several times with no response, Tony made his way to their bedroom. There, he found Sophie sitting on the side of the bed, looking confused. She said, "Poppa, I don't know what I'm supposed to do." Tony's heart fell. He realized with sadness that Sophie had progressed to a different stage in her illness. The transito-

> ry plateau to which he had adjusted had crumbled. After a brief period of self-pity and feeling defeated, he resolved to reinvent the routine to meet Sophie's current needs. From the recesses of his mind, he all of a sudden heard and then heard more clearly and then heard himself singing loudly, "Pick yourself up, dust yourself off, and start all over again."

Tony's triumph was due to his resiliency and ability to persist and gain control of both his actions and his emotions, in spite of adversity. Although these strengths may be part of his innate character, you can all learn and practice these important survival skills. You might also want to practice your singing.

COPING AND RESILIENCE

Caregiving can be a discouraging experience at times. We observe how some of you deal with stress with more resiliency than others. What are you doing that's different? You may have coped well and felt competent and self-confident before becoming a caregiver. Even if you temporarily lose faith in yourself, once you regain a sense of control over the situation, you recompose and cope again. You can adapt by acknowledging what it is you're facing and feeling and with that awareness, consciously change your negative thoughts, actions, and behaviors into something more productive. This, for example, is what Tony had to accomplish in order to feel he was coping effectively.

Your coping skills, thoughts, beliefs, and attitude about life can either help or hinder how you fare and how you handle the negative events that present themselves in your caregiving situation. To deal effectively and capably, it is essential that you be willing to change what is in your power to change. What can you alter? You can alter your negative attitudes and thoughts by modifying and reconstructing how you view and respond to stimuli in these circumstances. You do this by paying attention to how you're talking to yourself. What are you telling yourself? Are your thoughts critical, negative, and pessimistic? When we think negatively or pessimistically about our actions, failures, mistakes, or losses, we find ourselves depressed and in despair. You can change your thoughts as well as the way you react to and interact with provocations and irritants in your environment. Martin Seligman, clinical researcher and best-selling author, says, "Resilience in the face of challenges can be acquired." It is a skill that can be both taught and learned. Without a doubt, the course of Alzheimer's disease is difficult, but you can learn to change how you react and take control, thus developing optimism and hope.

Think about other challenging events you've experienced in your life. When adversity struck, how did you react? Is there a pattern? Do you tend to denigrate yourself and tell yourself that you're a loser, or insist that you cannot cope, or perceive yourself as weak? If you've convinced yourself that this is true, do you then throw your hands in the air and give up? What do you believe about yourself?

We've seen so many caregivers caught in the grip of despair turn things around by talking to themselves more encouragingly and also giving themselves permission to be just a little imperfect. The way you think about how you cope has significant repercussions. As Martin Seligman says, "optimism prompts us to change, while pessimism bids us to cower."

Our beliefs are very powerful. Our inner voices are louder and carry more weight than voices we hear externally—from friends, society, or parents for example. The consequences of our beliefs can either energize us (if they're positive) or depress us (if they're negative). When you have identified your negative belief, you can dispute its validity. Just as you can have a difference of opinion or a heated argument with another person, so, too, can you disagree with your faulty thinking. If you do so, you may very well find that you are blowing things out of proportion. Just because you hold this thought in your mind, does not make it true. The best thing to do is to take a time-out. Create some distance between yourself and this negative thought. Then proceed to seek evidence for the validity of the thought. How true is it? Think of situations over the course of your life where you have rallied and made an impact.

Can it be different? What thought might be more useful to you at this time? Is there an alternate way of viewing the situation? Can you see that just because you felt ineffective in one situation, this does not define you as a generally inadequate person? What can you do differently? How useful is it to hold this belief if the result is that you cave in? Instead of seeing the picture as all black or white, can you achieve a more balanced view?

Look at your particular situation and begin to figure out what it is you can change and what it is that you can control. It is when you gain control that you no longer feel helpless or hopeless. When you take action, your thoughts and emotions are influenced and transformed. Acting as your own agent optimizes self-esteem and gives meaning and hope to your life. You'll discover that instead of spiraling downward, you will feel motivated, encouraged, and strengthened, and more able to deal with the challenging situation more effectively. Even if you "mess up," you can often go back and undo what was done, or just move on. It is all up to you. You have many choices, and only you can make the decision about whether you will live your life with optimism or pessimism. We urge you to rally around hope and faith in your amazing human repertoire of untapped potential.

CHAPTER 5

Rallying the Troops: Family Reactions

Alzheimer's disease profoundly affects the patient, the spouse, and individual family members and the family unit. In some families, adult children, whether they live close to home or far away, may have a hard time accepting the reality that their parents are aging and becoming frail. Children, who have loved, respected, and looked up to their parent, are now faced with an emotional upheaval similar to the caregiver's, and denial may be even more powerful. They might continue to deny the behavioral changes that become apparent and are acknowledged by the caregiver as problematic or symptomatic. Even though sympathetic to these feelings, you, the caregiver, may feel unsupported as you contend with the practical and emotional issues at the onset of Alzheimer's. On the other hand, you may tend to shield your children from learning the reality about the illness for as long as possible.

Sylvia

Sylvia talked about her ambivalence in exposing Phil's Alzheimer's to their family.

> In the early stages of the disease, Phil often answered the phone and would converse briefly with the person on the other end. He sounded normal, and because his initial conversation was so coherent, it was often difficult to convince our children or other family members that he was in the early stages of Alzheimer's disease. I knew telephone contact was difficult for him. Shortly after Phil would answer the phone, I would see that confused look on his face, and he would abruptly end the conversation by saying something like, "Okay, honey, here's your mom," and he'd hand the phone over to me. It was a conundrum for me to decide how to handle the situation. I wanted to protect Phil and the children from this horrible reality, and yet I also wanted our family and friends to be aware of the situation with which I was dealing.

Occasionally it may be the children who begin to notice and acknowledge the early symptoms of Alzheimer's disease. They may share their observations and concerns with the well parent, who may not be ready to accept that something is indeed wrong. This was true in Angela's situation.

Angela

> My daughters were the first to communicate their suspicions about their dad to me, though at the time I was neither willing nor ready to agree with them. I was a pro at making excuses for Joe's behavior. My daughters continued

to insist that their father was not functioning competently, and I was getting more and more steamed at them. They wouldn't get off my case. Begrudgingly, I finally agreed to take Joe to a neurologist for a workup. Once the diagnosis of probable Alzheimer's was made, my daughters were relieved and their support allowed me to cope through my initial struggle. First I had to overcome my denial. Once I did, I was then able to explain his behavior to the rest of our family and friends. In fact, I was very open about it, telling my neighbors and other people with whom we came into contact. I believed that in telling everyone, they would, in turn, be forgiving and less offended by Joe's unusual behaviors. This was true in most instances. Boy, you really learn who your true friends are very quickly with this illness.

Mannie

Mannie had attended our support group for about a year when he approached me, asking to set up a family meeting for him and his daughters, who were having a hard time accepting their mother's decline. They were also very worried about Mannie.

When we met, Mannie's daughters tearfully explained how dearly they loved both of their parents and how difficult it was to see their mother, who had been the strength and backbone of the family, become helpless. They also expressed concern about their father's ability to cope. Since their mother had ruled the roost, her word was "law" and Mannie would go along happily with whatever she decided. They saw their dad as quite dependent on her and worried about his ability to care for himself and their mother. In addition, he had had cardiac bypass surgery a few years earlier, and they were concerned about his health and stamina. It was

> apparent at this meeting that Mannie felt supported and loved. In this safe setting, he and his daughters were able to talk openly about their hopes and fears for the first time. Mannie told his daughters what kind of help he thought he needed, and, in turn, they were able to make a plan the family could live with for the moment. It was a very simple plan. Mannie would continue with the primary care of his wife and attend the support group regularly. He reassured his daughters that caregiving was a job he wanted to take on, explaining that it was a way he could give back to his wife of sixty years, who had always taken such good care of him. His daughters would take turns visiting on alternate weekends. All of them supported the idea that Dad would bring in someone to help with the cooking and cleaning and stay with Mom, so he could get out a few days a week.

The outcome of this meeting was that the family began to feel more in control, more empowered, because now they were willing to work together and support each other. Despite their ongoing sadness and sense of loss, talking together in that environment that day also seemed to bring into reality their mother's decline. They were beginning to come to terms—together.

Taking into consideration the context and the history of relationships as well as the dynamics of the family itself is important. Considering how complex relationships can be in any family, whether family members have been loving and close or conflicted and distant, initiation into an understanding of this disease and an acknowledgment of the task at hand is an ongoing challenge.

As with Mannie and his daughters, you may need assistance in understanding how the dynamics in your family affect your willingness and ability to care compassionately for your spouse or parent. This knowledge is vital. We encourage you to reach out for support, whether in a group setting or individual counseling. Either or both of these options can strengthen family ties and enable the family to contend with the crisis of Alzheimer's disease.

If you feel at a loss as to how to seek appropriate outside help, your Alzheimer's Association is an excellent resource for finding a support group and/or selecting a psychotherapist familiar with the task of taking care of a loved one suffering from dementia. The goal is to get some help in understanding your response as well as your family's response to the illness and to determine a plan of action. It is okay to ask for help. In fact, it is more than okay. It is essential for your well-being and to maintain cohesion in your family.

CHAPTER 6

The Shell Without the Pearl: Transcending Loss

During these first stages of Alzheimer's disease, when the symptoms are subtle and erratic, the seeds are sown that will forever change the landscape of the marital relationship. This immutable transformation begins insidiously—perhaps a small disagreement, an angry word, an uncharacteristic insensitivity, or an inadvertent lapse of memory. These behaviors take place inconsistently but are aberrant enough to sap the foundations of the marriage.

Imperceptibly but inexorably, the relationship begins to change. The daily chitchat between spouses becomes more perplexing and exasperating as short-term memory and verbal skills deteriorate, making conversation a chore instead of a pleasant interaction. Tension develops as you begin to anticipate irrational interchanges. You're confronting challenging questions: What has happened to intelligent conversation? Why can we no longer make decisions together? Why do so many interactions involve acrimony instead of agreement? What happened to the respectful and loving discussions that we used to have? Why has my spouse become emotionally distant toward me?

Because of the continuing deterioration in the brain, due to Alzheimer's disease, conversations that necessitate the use of appropriate judgment, reason, memory, and emotion become an adversary, which can, in some relationships, undermine the partnership. Unfortunately, these abilities are lost fairly early during the onset of this dementing illness.

For many caregivers, this relationship has been a central and long-term interpersonal commitment often lasting thirty or more years. We have known several caregivers who have celebrated their sixtieth anniversaries! After so many years, it is as if you have a symbiotic union, a closeness, security, and, for some, a strong dependency on your mate as the "other half." By this time, you know each other so well that each could probably complete the other's sentences. A great sense of stability often develops out of that consistency and predictability, thus making the losses related to Alzheimer's that invade the relationship all the more profound.

LOSS OF MUTUALITY

Many relationships are characterized by a deep sense of love, compassion, and mutuality. As the disease progresses, these qualities in this marital context become one-sided. Mutuality and reciprocity are no longer possible as the Alzheimer's victim becomes more incapacitated by this illness. We have often heard caregivers remark that their relationship is now one-sided; they give and nothing comes back—no thanks, no gratitude, no smile of appreciation. In the following story, however, Paul was able to accept the one-sidedness of the relationship and continue on with compassion and optimism.

Paul

During every visit I made to Paul's home, he would tell me that it was not the major events of the marriage that he missed, it

> was the little things—the routine encounters of affection and devotion experienced in his marriage of forty years. Now they were just cherished memories. Paul reminisced, "Often, while Jane was cooking I would mischievously pull her apron strings. She would laughingly scold me and tell me what an awful pest I was. Her eyes would twinkle with playfulness. I also felt that she had a second sense about me. Jane seemed to know instinctively when I needed to be comforted. As soon as I walked through the door after a trying day at work, she would drop everything, and listen to my tale of woe, somehow knowing just the right words to use to soothe me."
>
> On one visit, as I arrived, Paul was walking Jane to her chair, supporting most of her weight. An old Benny Goodman tune was on the radio, and Paul began to dance with Jane, a delicate rag doll. "See, Mary," he said, "we can still dance." He was smiling though his eyes welled with tears.

It was the solidity of Paul and Jane's love that gave Paul strength to persevere through his wife's declining health. We are reminded that it is not only the monumental events of birth, death, and taxes that have cemented these relationships, but the ordinary day-to-day celebrations of being together. The joie de vivre, the spontaneity and well-being that contextualized the marital relationship, are a tremendous loss. It is the abiding memories and love Paul has for Jane that will sustain him.

LOSS OF PERSONALITY

Alzheimer's disease robs the victim of personality traits: a gentle manner, humor, kindness, intelligence, and patience that may have initially attracted you to your spouse. These traits are sometimes replaced by opposite, negative characteristics, such as aggression, moodiness, and irrationality. The observable changes in your spouse's personality are disheartening, and you begin to talk about the loss of the spouse you once knew.

In the following story, Yvette tried to master her disappointment and anger in the maddening metamorphosis she saw in her husband, Richard.

Yvette

> Richard was such a dear man. I always felt so blessed to have met and married such a kind and loving person. He was my best friend as well as my husband. I can't believe what I am about to say, but the truth is he has changed so much, that if I were to do this over again, I would never marry the man he is today. This dreadful disease has irrevocably changed his personality. He used to be tender, but he has become aggressive. He yells at me. The Rich I married never raised his voice to me, even when we squabbled. He has become so crude, and he used to treat me so respectfully. I feel as if I've lost my friend as well as my loving spouse, which makes taking care of him a true burden.

Yvette's situation is particularly poignant. When we fall in love and marry, the attraction is to the "person." We also develop a sense of security and comfort in the roles defined by that "personality." As Rich's personality diminished, caregiving became more difficult for Yvette. However, it is usually our memory of how this person used to be that gives us the strength to navigate new terrain and commit to caring for this stranger, who looks all too familiar.

In being able to work through her feelings of anger and disappointment so that she could feel better about caring for Rich, Yvette reached out for the support of her peers in the caregiver's group. From the outset of her new role as caregiver, as you will see throughout the book, the caregiver's support group was invaluable to her in all of the transitions she encountered with her husband's illness.

LOSS OF COMMUNICATION

Communication between human beings is a vital and complex process. In order for communication to be effective, it requires both a sender and a receiver. We use words and form sentences in order to send a verbal message to the receiver. Another powerful message is observed at the same time via our body language or nonverbal communication. We rely on our brains to perform myriad complex tasks that are needed for the message to be accurately received, deciphered, and sent. It is the brain that helps us to make sense of and interpret the sounds that we hear and even those we don't hear but observe while the message is being delivered. That is, we respond to both the verbal and nonverbal communiqué. All of these tasks function automatically and smoothly in a mind that is healthy. When brain function is impaired due to illnesses such as Alzheimer's disease, stroke, or Transient Ischemic Attacks (TIAs), for example, which ultimately damage the cortical areas involved in memory, language, and motor functions, these messages can no longer be interpreted or sent with accuracy. The patient may not understand what is being expressed, and even if he does, he may quickly forget due to memory problems. He may not be able to respond or react appropriately. Direct and respectful communication between two people becomes severely compromised. The toughest element for you to come to terms with is that normal everyday conversation in which you share your feelings and ideas, ask for what you want, or feel acknowledged begins to fade into oblivion. As the disease progresses, problems evolve with understanding the impaired person's attempts to converse with others, as well as our efforts to communicate directly to the patient. Not only does the Alzheimer's patient have difficulty making himself understood, but he also has trouble receiving, retrieving, and remembering what was said.

Carolyn

Carolyn was a newcomer to the support group; her husband, John, was in the early stages of Alzheimer's disease. She shared her aggravation about the loss of communication between John and herself and lamented about how their interactions had deteriorated. Tearfully, Carolyn told how their daily conversation had declined.

> In the past, John and I were able to discuss everything; however, these days this is no longer true. We used to have lively conversations about everything. John was so reasonable, fair, and flexible. Nowadays, we seem to argue about everything. He is so contrary and irrational. I try to reason with him, but that makes things worse. We hardly ever talk calmly about any topic. It can be as simple as my asking him if he'd like toast or cereal for breakfast. He will tell me that he already ate breakfast and will demand that I serve him lunch. Demand, mind you; he does not ask politely as he used to. I attempt to correct him and tell him we have not eaten breakfast yet. This is enough to cause him to explode. It only gets worse as the day goes on, and I just feel drained by the end of it.

It is also important to understand John's overreaction when Carolyn tries to reason with him about having already eaten breakfast. It is called a catastrophic reaction, which, simply put, means that the patient, due to the diminishing capacity of his brain, has an excessive emotional reaction, which is out of his control. He may become angry, upset, yell, strike out at you, or become depressed even when the situation may not seem to warrant such an extreme emotional reaction. You may be attempting to feed, clothe, or bathe your loved one and be confronted by an inappropriate overreaction. Understanding that this is part of the illness is important. It may also help you in dealing with these potentially exhausting situations to understand that there may be too much stimulation for the Alzheimer's victim, or too many choices offered that are upsetting and confusing.

It is important that you remain calm and reassure your loved one. Give simple instructions, go step by step, and explain in a soft voice what you are about to do. For example, if you're attempting to undress your partner, say, "I'm going to help you with your shirt." Then take it one step at a time. Think about what you do first when you take a shirt off. For example, you can say, "Put your hands up so that I can pull the shirt over your head." You can also demonstrate what it is you mean and even gently guide your loved one's arms upward. When this is done, then explain the next step: "Good. Now I am going to pull your shirt off." You can apply this to every situation, from eating to bathing and so on. Face your spouse and talk calmly and softly, with patience. Go slowly and be gentle. Don't argue or try to reason. If your loved one becomes fidgety or aroused, it is often a good idea to back off and wait a while before approaching him again.

Often, what you do not realize is your role in contributing to this negative interaction. By no means is this statement meant to blame or to be critical of you. It is merely to highlight how easy it is to be seduced into this pattern of continual and unproductive imbroglios. The following story illustrates this point.

Jane

With exasperation, Jane told the group how riled she was with her husband because of his constant bickering.

> I try to be patient with Mac. I explain everything to him. Mac will ask me for food just after we have eaten. I will explain to him that we just ate. He gets mad and demands something to eat. He accuses me of trying to starve him. If we go shopping, he insists on buying groceries that we already have at home. When I tell him we do not need whatever he is choosing to

> buy, he will cause a scene in the store just like a young child. I give in just so he will quiet down. What I really want to do is run out of the store and leave him there. I feel so embarrassed by his behavior. Last week, after I had planted some new seedlings in the garden, he went and pulled them out. I told him that he just ruined my garden and that he had not pulled out weeds, but little plants. He became so angry and then accused me of telling him that he was crazy. I simply do not know how to handle these altercations anymore. I am becoming so irritated that I am afraid of what I might say or do to him one of these days.

The group resonated with Jane's dilemma. They offered her words of sympathy and encouragement. Their solution was simple and practical, arising out of their all-too-familiar experiences with their spouses. They told Jane that it was she who would have to alter the way she spoke to her husband. They recommended that she not explain, or confront, or argue, or attempt to prove her point. Their suggestion was for Jane to try to distract him, acknowledge his feelings, agree with him, and just leave the room for a while until she had calmed down. It seemed that this was just what Jane was ready to hear. From the look of calm in her face, it seemed to have struck a chord within her.

When Jane returned to the support group the following week, she was delighted to inform the members that she had taken their advice and remarked on how smoothly the week had gone. She said she had not realized how much she was sabotaging their interactions with her determination to "help" Mac by explaining how wrong he was.

This is a very common scenario. You struggle to help your spouse understand what he or she has done incorrectly or what he or she ought to do. You explain, cajole, and attempt to reason with him. Before you know it, you're caught up in what becomes a battle where neither person wins because this is not a level playing field. By this time, you have become distraught, shaken, and overwhelmed by a sense of futility. Plus, aside from all this, you have fostered a catastrophic reaction, making the entire episode what can only be described as a folie à deux (a shared delusion). Often the behavior of an Alzheimer's patient is referred to as childish: "Oh, he's acting just like a child." The difference between a young child and an Alzheimer's patient is that the patient cannot change his behavior or learn new behaviors. This distinction is important to remember. We need to reemphasize that it is you, the caregiver, who must adjust to changes in the relationship by analyzing the problem and creatively modifying your reactions. Yes, it's not fair, but it is the only productive alternative.

Mannie

I used to become so angry with Rachel when she would undo the bed I had just finished making. She would take the comforter off, fold it, and take the pillows out of their cases. She would also empty the drawers and look for suitcases in which to pack her clothing. I was so impatient! I would become so incensed. I am ashamed to say, one day I yelled at her, "Rachel, how can you be so stupid? Can't you see that I have just made the bed? Get out of here." Then I felt remorseful and guilty. Thanks to the support group I was attending, I finally realized that it was not Rachel who was undoing the bed, but the disease that was compelling her to act this way. Once I could differentiate between Rachel and the behaviors due to the illness, I felt enormous relief and I could speak to Rachel with more patience and compassion. The behaviors were still very frustrating. Sometimes I would go into the kitchen, close the door, and pound on the table. Other times, realizing that it was really not important how the bed was made, or if it was made at all, I would just forget it. What seemed essential was to keep our relationship as respectful as it had once been. It was not an easy change to make since I was often riled up. However, when I looked into Rachel's eyes and saw fear and uncertainty, it was a cue to back off. These eyes clouded now

> by Alzheimer's are no longer the sparkling eyes of my lovely bride from years past, but they can still send a message to me and anchor my behavior.

It is essential for all of you to accept the fact that you will encounter all sorts of negative feelings. The nature of Alzheimer's is filled with ambiguity and guile. Give yourself permission to be angry, frustrated, resentful, and so on. It's natural and normal to experience negative emotions, because, after all, you are human, and expressing feelings is part and parcel of being a mere mortal. Don't make matters worse by berating yourself and then feeling guilty. Be kind and accepting of yourself. After all, you are doing the best you can in a very demanding situation with an intractable disease that can confound you and test your limits to a degree that you've never experienced before.

Loss of reasonable communication is a caregiver's common lament. However, once you fully comprehend the decline in ability to reason and short-term memory in the early stages of Alzheimer's, you can begin to alter the way that you communicate with your spouse. You may want to back down from always needing to be right or contradicting your spouse. Being right or wrong is often of little importance in the scheme of things. It is better to preserve his or her dignity and also to recognize the futility of engaging in any argument. Reasoning, explaining, teaching, and arguing are of no practical value and take a lot of otherwise useful energy.

LOSS OF PHYSICAL INTIMACY

Because it is a sensitive issue and regarded as extremely private and personal, the topic of physical intimacy is not one that is often discussed openly. However, we recognize the importance sexual intimacy plays in a healthy relationship and the validity of its loss. Intimacy includes both emotional and physical closeness: giving and receiving love, intercourse, affectionate touching, holding hands, fondling, caressing, hugging, and even conversation. Due to damage and deterioration in the brain, the desire for physical intimacy goes awry. It may intensify, decrease, or disappear. The decorum and emotions of adult intimacy are no longer understood by the Alzheimer's patient. However, the desire or longing by the patient to feel loved does not disappear. The caregiver is faced with another loss and another dilemma. The choice to continue having sexual intimacy is subjective, but you do have a choice.

With great sadness as well as embarrassment, caregivers have spoken about the loss of physical and sexual intimacy. Sylvia confessed to me privately that her sexual relationship with Phil had deteriorated. She joked a little but was disconsolate as she mourned this significant loss in their relationship.

Sylvia

> The one activity I miss and long for is sex with my hubby. I bet you're surprised that an old lady of seventy-eight was still enjoying an active sex life. Phil and I always had a fulfilling intimate relationship. We would often just reach out for each other at night in bed, to hold each other. I felt content in his arms, and I miss having them around me, cuddling and making love, or simply holding me. He doesn't know how to meet those needs anymore.

Nate

Nate spoke of his regrets that sex was no longer a part of his relationship with Flora.

> I still feel very attracted to my wife and continue to have a desire for sexual intimacy. However, since she is so confused, I fear that I would be taking advantage of her to satisfy my own

needs, and she wouldn't understand what was going on. Also, her behaviors are so childlike, it just would not seem right!

Some caregivers, who have had active sexual lives with their spouses, express guilt or anxiety about continuing to have feelings of arousal. It is important to celebrate the fact that the relationship once had passion and to understand that experiencing such desires is normal. Losing this vital part of the relationship is very profound.

With Alzheimer's disease, inappropriate sexual behavior can also become manifest and difficult for the caregiver. On my first visit with Hannah and Max, I had more than a secondhand experience with Max's sexual behavior.

Hannah

As Hannah greeted me at the front door, I saw her husband, a dapper little older man, approaching. Before Hannah could even introduce me, he grabbed me and gave me a big wet kiss on the mouth. A little startled, I broke away from his grasp, but poor Hannah was completely mortified. She apologized, and immediately I suspected that this behavior was probably a repetitive problem with which she dealt. We proceeded to the living room where Hannah sat down in what seemed to be her usual chair, and I sat at one end of the sofa. Max joined us after a bit and sat at the other end of the sofa. As I was interviewing Hannah, I noticed out of the corner of my eye that Max was slowly creeping closer and closer to me, and before I knew it, he was right next to me with his hand on my thigh. Hannah immediately escorted him out of the room, and I heard her turning on the television in another location. After Hannah recomposed, it was hard for us not to find this whole scenario extraordinarily funny, but I also had great sympathy for her. She sat back down and told me of similar incidences.

> Max won't leave me alone. He keeps grabbing at me and wanting to touch me in private places. I find it so degrading and even abhorrent. He does this several times a day, whether I'm busy cooking or cleaning or trying to watch the news. It doesn't even end there. When I took him to his doctor's appointment last week at the VA Hospital, he tried to embrace one of the nurses. I was really humiliated. I'm afraid to go shopping or anywhere with Max now because I don't know when he will become sexually inappropriate, or with whom. Max would never, never act this way before he developed Alzheimer's.

For Hannah, feeling abused and disrespected compounded the loss of intimacy and added more stress to her everyday life. Due to the brain damage caused by Alzheimer's disease, Max became disinhibited, which is not an unusual behavior; however, neither is it very common. Over time, her frustration intensified until she mastered redirecting Max's inappropriate sexual behavior. Hannah learned to distract her husband by offering him something to eat, turning on the TV, or taking him for a drive in the car. Hannah also spoke with Max's neurologist, who placed him on medication that decreased his disruptive behavior, allowing her to resume taking him out in public. In doing these things, Hannah was able to gain control over Max's inappropriate behavior while still preserving his self-esteem as well as her own. (See more about the loss of intimacy in Part 2, The Middle Stage.)

LOSS OF PARTNERSHIP

Each of you, due to the unique contextual as well as historical factors that define your partnership, experiences losses differently. The degree and intensity of the loss will vary as well. If the marriage has been long, satisfying, and congenial, the losses are perceived with greater sadness and grief. In marriages that have been fraught with discord or are more recent and without the long history of commitment, feelings of loss are less pervasive. In those cases sometimes the experience of the decline in the spouse is met with more resentment and anger. If the marital relationship had been acrimonious, caregivers may be tormented by feelings of guilt and shame as they struggle to remain compassionate when caring for their spouse affected with Alzheimer's disease. Loss of the partnership becomes secondary to the loss of freedom, feelings of entrapment and obligation to the inevitable confinement and restrictions of being a caregiver.

LOSS OF SENSE OF BELONGING: ISOLATION

According to Dr. Rudolf Dreikurs, noted child psychiatrist and author of *Psychodynamics, Psychotherapy, and Counseling*, "The fundamental desire of every human being is to belong, to have status in the group of which he is a part. He can fulfill himself only within the group. Without belonging he is lost and life becomes meaningless."

One of the first changes that is both self- and other imposed, is isolation. In your routine family and social interactions, for example, at the golf club, church coffee hour or communal dinner, you may notice subtle rejection. Like Alzheimer's disease, isolation has a subtle beginning. You may also feel embarrassed by your spouse's repetitiveness, forgetfulness, or ill manners as you abide the disapproving glances, real or imagined, of your companions. In addition, some Alzheimer's patients may become reluctant to fraternize, because they are aware of the memory losses and changes in their behavior and wish to preserve their waning self-esteem. It is important to understand that the experience for the patient of being in large groups can be confusing and disorienting, resulting in the desire to withdraw. Finding these occurrences difficult, caregivers often begin to detach from social situations that once gave them meaning and a sense of belonging.

In some families, it is not uncommon for adult children to withdraw and detach from their ill parent. Changes in the image of their parent as the strong, supportive, and loving role model are difficult to reconcile at this time. Seeing the parent become frail and childlike is painful. When this happens, not only does the healthy parent become isolated, but also the children forsake their ties to their family. We encourage you and your children to be patient with each other and continue to communicate with clarity and consistency about the feelings you are experiencing. In reality, in some families this may not be an easily accomplished task.

Edith

> Our two sons live close by, and when Edward was diagnosed with Alzheimer's, I thought their proximity would be a real blessing. But when Edward began to show changes in his personality and competency, our sons seemed to find excuses not to spend time with us. Even though they worked hard during the week, on the weekend, they no longer came over to watch the football game with their dad, nor did they run out to the hardware store together as they had routinely in the past. I was feeling hurt and confused by their excuses and their absence. Instead of feeling supported, I felt so alone.

Edith and I discussed the possibility that her sons were having a difficult time facing the illness and that perhaps their denial was the reason for their disappearing act. We spoke of the importance of communicating with her sons, not only about her hurt feelings, but also about their feelings in coming to terms with their father's illness. We agreed that she should tell them how important and necessary it is for her and for them to continue to participate in their father's life. The boys had been very close to their father, and Edith felt that it was crucial for them to maintain a strong bond with their dad through his illness. She did not want them to live with regret or self-recrimination after their father's death.

Because of their reticence to come over, Edith felt isolated and neglected by her sons. She missed their company and their family time together and feared that the family was disintegrating. She worried that she would not have their support in making major decisions that she and her husband could no longer make together. Edith needed some time to think about what we had discussed and whether she could be completely forthcoming with her sons about all of this. This might be difficult. A suggested recourse would be to seek the help of a professional, one who could get to the family's unspoken fears and repressed feelings in a safe setting. However, Edith bit the bullet and called her sons and told them of her hurt and confusion over their behavior. She also told them plainly that she needed their help. This took a lot of courage, and at first, her sons both denied there was anything underlying their absence. But the conversation struck a cord and they began to visit regularly. At first they admitted that it felt awkward and they didn't know what to say or how to handle their dad. Edith said, "Just be yourself." She gave them articles to read and generally was more open herself in discussing their father's situation and her feelings with them. Her husband was so happy to see his boys. They, as a family, were coming to terms with Alzheimer's by sharing their grief and showing compassion and acceptance, both of their upsetting feelings and the tragic regression of their dad.

Jane

Jane's experience of isolation involved the lack of support and validation from her siblings. They simply didn't seem to understand how demanding it was to be taking care of an ill husband.

> Mac has been ill for some time now. I know that I am depressed and it is not fun to talk with me at times. However, I feel so hurt and angered by my sister and brother's attitude. They live out of town—one is in Texas and the other is in Minnesota. When I complain about how much of a prisoner I feel in my own home, and how difficult it has become to go anywhere with Mac, they tell me to get on with my life and

> urge me to leave him alone when I go out. They think I am babying him too much. I long for words of comfort and compassion, and I fear that their attitude is distancing us. I feel resentful and alone. Even though I send them articles about Alzheimer's disease to read, they seem to have no appreciation for how difficult daily life can be with an Alzheimer's patient. I sometimes think they still want to believe Mac is the same gregarious, capable guy they've known for years. We used to have so much fun. After the war, we were dirt poor but the four of us could just spend a whole evening playing pinochle, listening to the radio, and laughing at who knows what into the wee hours.

In sharing this vignette with her support group, Jane received understanding nods from some members who were experiencing similar disappointments and lack of understanding from their relatives. She was definitely not alone. The group's response was both validating and reassuring to her. One member suggested that she keep sending her siblings literature about Alzheimer's disease. Another said that Jane should extend an invitation for them to visit. This way, they would be able to see firsthand what she was going through. Very often caregivers feel disenfranchised, invisible. Many caregivers feel as if they are shackled, imprisoned—and find that few people concede that they are indeed in a very difficult situation. There is no better path to enlightenment than spending twenty-four hours in the shoes of the caregiver, or at least alongside of her. Members of the group urged the caregiver to leave for a few hours, or for the day, leaving the care of the patient in the hands of the visiting relatives. This "hands-on" experience would be very reinforcing. Jane was willing to give this invitation to visit a try. She truly wanted and needed her siblings' love, understanding, and support.

In the support group, caregivers also commiserate about the isolation they endure as they deal with the loss of contact with their friends. Sometimes the disconnection is self-imposed, and at other times it is the friends who take flight.

Bill told his story to the group with sadness, but without any bitterness in his voice.

Bill

I've deliberately withdrawn from socializing with certain friends. I made a conscious decision not to place my wife in situations that are uncomfortable for us or for our friends. You might ask why I decided to retreat. Well, quite honestly, I couldn't tolerate the obvious sorrow our friends felt for us. I could see the pity on their faces, and I was concerned that Hazel would sense their sympathy. I simply didn't want anyone adding to the burden we were already carrying. Thankfully, however, there are a few stubborn friends who have not allowed me to quit on them.

Betty

Elliot and I moved from our home in Michigan to a large retirement community in Southern California. We were very excited and eagerly anticipated this new adventure.

At first, we appreciated that everyone seemed as interested as we were in remaining active participants in our golden years. Most of our activities centered around the club and from that resource new friendships developed. I felt accepted and comfortable enjoying the companionship they provided. When my husband began to show subtle signs of Alzheimer's disease, I noticed with acuity the undermining of our social life. In the larger group activities—the club happy hour, the Sunday brunch—my husband often repeated stories, and his social skills were awkward and embarrassing. I was aware of the quizzical looks that our friends would direct toward Elliot and me and became quite sensitive to what I describe as "a subtle discrimination." At the club,

> bridge and golf were taken very seriously, and as Elliot became less competent and distracted, I withdrew from these activities before suffering the embarrassment of possibly being asked to leave. Most hurtful for me was the realization that friends had stopped calling to invite us to join them.

One reason for this rejection could have been that these folks were relatively new friends, lacking the history that forms "through thick and thin" bonds of friendship. Possibly, people withdrew because there is often a stigma attached to the apparent senescence (the forgetfulness, confusion, disorientation, and waning mental abilities of the demented patient) observed in Alzheimer's disease. Many times people simply feel awkward and uncomfortable, and don't know what to say to the demented person. Or, they could be frightened, as the situation may stir up subjective feelings of fear about their own aging and mortality. Many friends, old or new, do not fully comprehend the childlike behaviors and may be embarrassed and believe that their own reputation, through their association with that couple, could be besmirched, and therefore they withdraw. It is also likely that friends may be reluctant to openly confront or question any of the unusual and conspicuous behaviors they observe. Whatever the reason for the withdrawal, the hurtful actuality is that the avoidance of the friendship leaves caregivers feeling estranged, rejected, and lonely.

Since explaining your spouse's behavior may be difficult and awkward, it is you who might unwittingly participate in avoidant behavior, feeling insecure about how to address the truth of your spouse's decline and loss of abilities. On the other hand, your friends might be reluctant to broach the subject, because they don't know how you will react to their queries. Inadvertently, often acting out of this fear and ignorance, friends may cause the caregiver and patient to feel left out, shamed, and disgraced as well. We would heartily encourage you to take the initiative and openly have a conversation about Alzheimer's with these friends. Educate them, for this could solve this circular conundrum, which leads to isolation. Try to understand that the stigma is not directed toward you or your spouse, but rather toward the misunderstood, aberrant behaviors that are caused by Alzheimer's disease.

As you will learn, it is you, the caregiver, who must initiate the conversations or actions to facilitate change. Thus it was with Betty. After feeling frustrated for a long time, she courageously decided to cover her hurt, swallow her pride, and call two of the women with whom she felt the closest to come over for coffee. Once they all sat down, Betty came right out with it. She told them that Elliot had Alzheimer's disease and asked them if they had any questions she might be able to answer about his illness. This gave her friends the opportunity to be educated about Alzheimer's disease and voice any apprehension. Then she talked openly about how the illness was affecting her and changing her relationships. She didn't want them to feel sorry for her or guilty; instead she wanted to present a realistic picture and let the chips fall where they may, with the hope that she would not be completely rejected. The choice was now theirs. Could these two friends develop empathy, let go of their fears, and be willing to remain involved in the friendship? Would they make concessions because of Elliot's illness that would still allow Betty some participation in the social circle? We learned that only one of the two women remained a friend to Betty, but it became an invaluable, cherished friendship.

Jane

Jane expounded upon her feelings of isolation. She felt comforted and a little surprised by what happened in the support group.

> My husband and I moved from Ohio to California about one and a half years ago. Six months afterward, my husband was diagnosed with Alzheimer's disease. I never had a chance to make meaningful friendships. All of our old friends are in Ohio, and although we keep in touch by phone, it's very difficult to talk about Mac and our situation because he's always present. When I'm on the phone, he won't leave me alone. He wants to know who I'm talking to. He tries to hang up the phone, par-

> ticularly if he even thinks I'm talking about him. So, my conversations are stilted and disjointed. Anyway, long-distance communication is not the same as being able to have friends visit or pop in and talk over a cup of coffee.

Jane paused and reflected on what she had just said. Then she exclaimed:

> Do you know this is the first time I have spoken so openly about how lonely I feel and how Mac's illness is affecting me? It's such a relief to be able to share what I feel with people who really understand.

Every member of the group was sympathetic. Each individual could understand, from his or her own experiences, Jane's feelings of loneliness. On the other hand, Jane left the support group that day feeling a lot lighter. It seemed as if an enormous burden had been lifted off her shoulders. Her spirits rose and she was touched by the understanding and kindness offered to her by the members of the group. Becoming part of a support group helps you feel a profound sense of belonging and identification with others who are in the same boat as you are.

During this crisis in your life, there is a great need for support from friends and family who can provide encouragement and help you hang in there. When they "disappear," they take with them the pleasures involved in social contacts and the confidence you've had in your place in society. Until you feel the security of a supportive network of friends and family, you may feel disenfranchised, isolated, unsettled. The onus is on you to drive this evolution, which will result in strengthening bonds of friendship and finding a sense of belonging and connection within a new social context.

As always, time is also the reliable healer. If you are patient, the knowledge of your loved one's illness will be fully realized over time by reluctant or disbelieving family and friends.

In "The Beginning Stage" we originate the journey of remarkable caregivers, like you, who have begun to navigate through the twists and turns of the discovery of Alzheimer's disease and its impact on your life and those of your loved ones. Although frightened and floundering at first, through education, experience, and social support, you begin to acknowledge the disease. You begin to accept your feelings and become less critical and judgmental of yourself concerning their presence. This allows you to reach deep inside yourself to find the hope and courage to move forward on this unpredictable course while retaining your self-worth and that of your loved one.

DISCOVERING THE PARADOX OF CAREGIVING

It is evident that it is within the varied losses you suffer that you discover the ultimate paradox of caregiving. While your need for staying connected, mutuality, communication, sexual intimacy, and belonging are intact, your patient has dispensed with all. Aaron Alterra, in his book *The Caregiver: A Life with Alzheimer's*, discusses this very paradox when, in reference to his wife, he says, "Presence is what counts. You can understand with what hesitation I say it would not be traumatic for her to lose a child or grandchild, . . . If I disappear, she will not have difficulty getting used to my absence. I keep coming back to that astonishing idea: If I am no longer present, it will not take Stella long to get used to it."

The nature of what the patient has lost, the ability to express appropriate emotion, which distinguishes us as human beings, is not in itself an emotional event for the patient. Paradoxically, you are deeply grieved and mourn the tragic loss of emotion and expression in your spouse and therefore epitomize what they have lost. As Alterra points out, while you continue to feel empathy, sorrow, the need for intelligent and significant connection and communication, your spouse's abilities are compromised. In fact, what you yearn for and what is no longer available to you in your relationship seems to hardly be missed by your loved one. You miss conversation. You have a hard day and would perhaps love to hear some consoling words, but the patient no longer has the capability of understanding your needs or the appropriate emotional response of offering sympathy.

You struggle to remain connected to your loved one, differentiating the patient from the disease, in order to protect against personal affront. You learn how to depersonalize the indifferent behavior. You eventually find an equilibrium that allows you to love and nurture your patient and yet live your own life to the fullest.

These first encounters with Alzheimer's disease include multiple losses, bereavement, and deprivation, and cover a wide range of emotions. Caregivers describe feeling sad, angry, confused, lonely, fearful, resentful, helpless, and overwhelmed. We would like to stress that these feelings are normal and encourage you to accept that this is so and not burden yourself by engaging in the struggle against natural human reactions. After all, an uninvited, cataclysmic interloper has intruded upon your life. As the disease progresses and you come to terms with the irreversible changes, you will gain control, confidence, and mastery.

PART TWO

THE MIDDLE STAGE

CHAPTER 7
Coming to Terms

Sylvia

Sylvia, who had been a spunky, active, and carefree woman, initially struggled with her forced role of caregiver when Phil, her husband of forty-six years, became ill. Before the onset of the illness, Sylvia had enjoyed tending to her garden, socializing with her friends, and playing the organ at church on Sundays. These pleasurable and rewarding activities had gradually ceased due to the demanding nature of Alzheimer's. The role of caregiver was especially difficult for Sylvia because, according to her, up until now, Phil had taken care of everything. He had been completely responsible for the finances, upkeep of their automobiles and the house, and had even bought the groceries. She had enjoyed his attentiveness and love as well as the security that this long and happy relationship had given her. Now Phil was becoming increasingly incompetent, and as his abilities deteriorated, so, too, in her own way, did Sylvia's. Having lost her spunk and spontaneity and ceased her activities with friends, she became sad and morose at times. Moreover, Sylvia was terribly dismayed when she found herself engulfed by anger. She was reticent to share her strong feelings with the support group, until one day, in an uncharacteristic fit of rage, her words tumbling onto one another, she poured out her long-pent-up feelings.

> Everything Phil does exasperates me. He moves my books, my purse, and my keys from place to place. I have yet to find the channel changer. He put the sink stopper in the toaster oven and turned it on. The stopper shriveled to almost nothing. He cut the cord on the radio. The battle of the bath continues every night. He becomes hostile and almost physically abusive when I try to remove his underpants, yelling, "And what do you think you are doing?" He laughs inappropriately and he talks gibberish, which unnerves me, and I do not know how to respond.

Shrugging her shoulders and shaking her head, Sylvia, her face wrenched with despair and tears welling up in her dark brown eyes, continued.

> Ohh! Just talking about it infuriates me, I'm angry with him so much of the time. I also feel so depressed and trapped. I could go on and on telling you of all the things he does to tick me off, but what good would it do? I really need some help.

Sylvia gasped for air and eventually let out a long sigh. As usual, the participants in the support group sprang to the rescue. They nodded their heads in empathic agreement and commiserated about how they, too, had experienced many of the same ordeals and feelings. Some attempted to console Sylvia by assuring her that these behaviors would not last very long. Some reminded Sylvia that it was the disease in Phil's brain that was making his behavior so uncontrollable. Others offered advice, suggesting that Sylvia look for someone to stay with Phil or that she consider sending him to a day-care program, so that she could continue to enjoy some of her old activities.

Nate, on the other hand, recalling his own experience with his wife, encouraged her to try and enjoy what Phil was still capable of doing well. He explained that he, too, had been pushed to the limits by these very behaviors and still had continued to fight the disease tooth and nail. One day, on the brink of cracking, he realized his continual dueling was useless and nothing was changing for the better. His triumph, he told Sylvia, was paradoxically when he was able to comprehend that he had come up against a disease that was intractable, unyielding, and unconquerable. The effect of this insight allowed him to consciously begin to separate the illness and it's effect on the behaviors of his wife from who his wife was and had always been to him. She was, after all, the victim of Alzheimer's disease. He had to mellow out and relinquish his stubborn belief that he could lick this thing. Instead, to cope and to feel useful, he would practice being a mediator between the illness and his wife. In doing so he was able to accept the negative behaviors with less immediate, reactive anger and more resilience.

Having had the unspoken permission to "let it out" in this safe arena and receiving unwavering support, Sylvia took a deep breath and continued with a more relaxed expression on her face.

> Thank you all. Nate, as you were speaking, what came to mind was how important it is to protect our loved one's dignity and to acknowledge how vulnerable they are. As I think of Phil, I realize how much I value his sweet, good side. You know, he still does little thoughtful things for me. He will pick up anything that I drop, and I so appreciate that, because bending is hard for me with my bad knees. He thanks me for everything. He doesn't complain about anything and is usually in good spirits. Gosh, I do feel lousy for having blown my stack like that. I'm finding it so difficult to acknowledge what is happening to Phil.

Sylvia's story reveals that coming to terms with the complex drama of Alzheimer's disease is extraordinarily challenging.

THE IMPORTANCE OF ACQUIRING COPING SKILLS

When you get that "gut sense" realization that you are reckoning with a disease that is uncompromising, unalterable, and mercurial, it's easy, natural, and very common to be filled with despair and begin to feel helpless. This attitude will not be an ally in your relationship with your loved one, with the disease, or with yourself. Caregiving is inundated with unexpected obstacles and hindrances. That is the nature of Alzheimer's disease. It behooves you to develop the coping skills you need so that you will not feel outmaneuvered, but capable and competent in dealing with it. To develop mastery and become adroit in managing the illness, your patient, and yourself takes both willingness to change your way of coping and effort on your part. This requires that you redirect the negative energy toward developing skills that increase your level of competence. It's all about how you talk to yourself; especially what you tell yourself with respect to your competence and worth in the context of being a caregiver. For example, if you believe that you will never cope or that you don't have what it takes to feel competent, you will be more likely to struggle more than you need to.

MANAGING YOUR ATTITUDES AND THOUGHTS

Remember beliefs and thoughts, although very loud, powerful, and persuasive in our minds, are not set in stone. They are also not always correct or rational. The following are some questions you can ask yourself about the benefits of changing your attitude and thoughts.

- What will I gain?
- If I think and act positively, how will this help my loved one?
- What will change for me?
- What is my belief about myself as a caregiver?
- What is the consequence of this belief?
- If I dispute or argue with this belief, what do I learn about the situation and myself?
- If I continue thinking like this, or reacting the way I do, how will this benefit both my loved one and myself?

When you acquire control over your situation, instead of a wavering self-esteem, your ego will be strengthened. Learn what it is that you can or can't control. For instance, you can neither control your spouse's behavior nor the disease. But you will discover that what you can control is your attitude and how you choose to respond. You can decide how you will act and what you will do in various situations. Remember, however, that you are human and not expected to be on top of the situation 100 percent of the time. Little steps, little moments of accomplishment are illuminating, enriching, and serve to reduce your anxiety. Some of you may find changing thoughts and behaviors easier to do than it is for others. However, don't despair. Changing your thoughts and beliefs is a skill that can be taught by a competent cognitive-behavioral therapist or by reading and educating yourself. There are many books that have been published, to guide caregivers on how to effectively manage your loved one's difficult behaviors. We want to continue to focus and concentrate on guiding you in increasing your understanding and awareness of your emotional reactions and their repercussions on you, your loved one, and others.

In this section of the book, the discussion and stories will focus on emotions experienced by other caregivers, who, like you, are dealing with the challenging and frustrating behaviors of their spouses now, in the middle stage of Alzheimer's disease.

MIDDLE-STAGE BEHAVIORS

Increasing memory loss, confusion, and shortened attention span are general characteristics of the middle stage of Alzheimer's disease. More specifically, your spouse may exhibit a decreased memory of recent events, such as a recent visit by a friend, or relevant personal information, such as his or her phone number. Orientation to time and place is compromised. Your loved one may forget how to get to familiar places or be unable to understand time of day in the context of the passage of time.

You may observe that your patient has difficulty in concentrating, organizing thoughts logically, or finding the right words to express what he or she is thinking. Your loved one may avoid complex tasks, withdraw from challenges, and try to cover for inability to verbalize by making up words to fill the gaps. Concurrently, you may notice a decreased ability to read, write, and calculate numbers.

Physically, your patient may have decreased motor skills and present with mild twitching or muscle jerks. He or she may become restless, particularly in the late afternoon. In the literature, this phenomenon is referred to as "sundowning."

Often more egregious to you are noticeable changes in your loved one's personality. You may encounter suspicion, silliness, irritability, lack of impulse control, and fixed ideas about unreal incidents. A flattening affect in facial expression may be discernable, and your loved one may no longer be able to connect with you with the same sensitivity or emotionality as he or she had in the past.

YOUR ROLE IN ACCOMMODATING TO THE MIDDLE STAGE

Commensurate to the changes in your loved one in the middle stage, your role also is altered. You will need to take on more responsibility, and care will begin to revolve around the clock as brain function further deteriorates an vgnd the patient's need for hands-on assistance in the activities of daily living (ADL) increases. You will need to assist your spouse in carrying out tasks such as dressing, eating, or brushing his or her teeth in the correct order. Tasks that have previously seemed automatic will now become a puzzle to the patient. For example, when you brush your teeth, there is usually a simple order: take the toothbrush out of the holder, reach for the toothpaste, uncap it, put a line of it on your toothbrush, recap the toothpaste, wet your brush, put the brush in your mouth, brush, and rinse. This activity alone can become too complicated for the Alzheimer's patient, who no longer knows how to sequence actions using the correct steps.

You will need to learn how to direct and take charge of necessary daily functions and yet allow your patient to maintain as much independence as possible. With dressing, for example, you could lay out clothing in the correct sequence in which one would put the items on: underwear on top, followed by pants and sweater, with socks and shoes last, and then allow your patient to dress him- or herself.

In the middle stage, at times memory losses are ambiguous and difficult to evaluate. Because competence in memory and other activities is uneven—one moment your loved one may appear to be quite well, even back to normal, and at another he may appear less capable than ever—your hopes soar and then, just as quickly, are dashed. You may be further frustrated when your loved one distorts the truth or fabricates stories. It is essential to understand that your spouse does this as a way of preserving his dignity and sense of self-worth, and possibly to hide his fears as he becomes insecure with the awareness that he is losing more of himself.

You notice that your loved one can no longer initiate any activities or tell you what he or she needs. His or her ability to find the right words, or to reason, or to understand, is by now severely compromised. Your loved one may not be able to make choices. However, if he or she still can, it is advisable to limit the choices: "Would you like to eat or dress now?" Eventually, you will need to direct an activity without giving a choice. For example, "It's time for lunch now."

It is probable that during this stage you'll need to accommodate symptoms such as delusions or hallucinations, repetitive behaviors or questions, less awareness of surroundings or lack of recognition of familiar people or places. Changes in mood can be mercurial and unpredictable. Sleep patterns may be altered, and sundowning or agitated behavior might become problematic. If these behaviors become unmanageable over time, your patient's physician may recommend an appropriate medication to modify the symptoms.

CHAPTER 8

Confronting the Demons: Your Emotional Reactions to the Middle Stage

Thinking again about Sylvia's story (Chapter 7), her strong and volatile reaction during this stage of Alzheimer's disease is not unusual. Caregivers' stories will illustrate that in the middle stage of the disease you will find yourself increasingly burdened with the care of your loved one. As your patient needs more from you, you must take caution against depleting all of your emotional and physical energy. The patient may push your buttons and try your patience to the limit. Other negative feelings, such as anger and frustration, may increase in intensity. You may find yourself more isolated as you cope with the twenty-four-hour-a-day demands of your spouse. This is the norm. As you learn how other caregivers have dealt with various situations as well as with their emotions, like them, you will find yourself succeeding and mastering the obstacles you confront with less reaction, a sense of control, and preservation of your health.

The following group meeting demonstrates some of the caregivers' common feelings, frustrations, and reactions resulting from the behavior of their patients in the middle stages. In order to normalize the gamut of emotions experienced by the caregivers, especially those who were uncomfortable verbalizing their negative sentiments, the question was asked, "What is your gut reaction to the question, 'What's really driving you up the wall in caring for your loved one?'" A number of hands went up. Participants were eager to describe the difficult behaviors that had thrown them off balance.

> Yvette, obviously irritated, blurted out, "Richard drives me crazy with his repetitive stories and questions. I have no patience with him when he can't find the right words or make sense when he talks. I've learned never to tell him ahead of time what we are going to do, because he becomes anxious and paces and asks over and over again, "When are we going?" After thirty minutes of this, I'm ready to scream.
>
> Bill, in a booming and resentful tone, described his difficulty coping with Hazel's mood swings. "I never know what's going on with Hazel anymore. One minute she's up. Next minute she's down. She's cheerful and then she's teary. Sometimes she gets mad over nothing. I always thought I knew her so well. Adjusting to her mood swings is so arduous. I simply don't know what to do or say to fix things. Quite frankly, I'm stymied."
>
> Impatient to speak, Carolyn burst in, "John used to have such a mild temperament, and now he seems to have no self-control. I'm afraid of him at times. He's no longer interested in bathing and cannot dress himself. Sometimes he's combative when I approach him to help or even suggest that he do something."
>
> Sylvia shuddered as she described one of her husband's scary behaviors: "I find it so creepy when Phil hallucinates. Mostly he sees bugs and other people. He hands me the 'bugs' he catches and gets upset if I don't take them from him, or if I tell him there is nothing there. The bugs really bug me. Excuse the pun. It used to be disconcerting and confusing when he'd ask me to pour coffee for his dead mother or call his deceased

sisters or brothers. Now, although it takes superhuman patience, I'm learning to accommodate all those people he's invited to live with us. His focus on bugs, however, still makes me shudder."

"My Joan still knows who I am," Steve began, "but the other day, much to my embarrassment, when our best friends, Mabel and Pete, were visiting, she kept confusing them with other friends and even our insurance salesman. She actually told Pete we didn't need any more life insurance. This is not the first time she failed to recognize familiar faces, but it was the first time it got to me."

Nate, with a baffled expression on his face, added, "For a long time I continued to believe that Flora was able to read. Last night, much to my surprise, I realized that the page she was supposedly reading, was the same one she had turned to when she first opened the book. I asked her what she was reading. I was crushed to discover that she had no recognition of the content and had been sitting there with her gaze fixed on the same page all afternoon. I just didn't want to believe it. I can't tell you how much I miss her candor, her sense of humor and intelligent discussions."

DENIAL

Because of the ambiguity of the diagnosis, "possible/probable Alzheimer's disease," many caregivers struggle with their denial. Although denial is often portrayed as negative, it can also serve a positive function. Denial can be viewed as an ally determined to protect you from confronting a painful reality until you have mustered up enough inner strength to deal with the situation. When you use a defense mechanism such as denial, for example, it is not so much that you are unaware of the reality of the diagnosis, but that when you project that reality into the future it becomes both too painful and scary for you to acknowledge at the time the diagnosis is made. When you are able to gain a sense of control and can plan, organize, and make decisions that effectively impact your future, you will become less frightened. When you acquire a sense of competence in handling both your reactions and your patient's symptoms, you will be able to transition into accepting the reality that at first overwhelmed you. Once this stage is achieved, you will then be able to let go of denial and come to terms with or meet head on the challenges of Alzheimer's disease. Each of you will transcend denial at your own pace—it is a process that cannot be rushed. Denial, however, becomes problematic when it interferes with your judgment or ability to manage your spouse and the varied and complex situations involved in caregiving.

Veronica

Veronica's story provides an excellent example of problematic denial. Her face pale and voice strained, she spoke about her husband, Zeke's, disconcerting behavior.

> We can no longer socialize with friends down at the clubhouse. I'm constantly humiliated because Zeke repeatedly asks the same questions and persists in telling the same stories. I think he is doing this to embarrass me. He never liked going to these club events anyway.
>
> He seems to want me to do more and more for him. Sometimes he doesn't eat his dinner or he picks up his meat in his fingers. Does he expect me to feed him? Zeke will not take his medications. I put them on the counter for him. I leave notes telling him when to take them. I remind him constantly. I'm doing all of this for him, and he does diddlysquat for me. I get so worked up talking about this, it convinces me all the more that he's lazy, selfish, and feeling sorry for himself.

Veronica was obviously unable to accept her husband's illness, and her denial made it inevitable that she would take his behaviors personally. Her intense denial became problematic when she said she would not be responsible for giving Zeke his medication. It took several months for members of the group to help Veronica understand that her husband's behaviors were a result of a brain disease, and that he truly had a memory problem and could not be trusted to remember to take his medication without her assistance. Her progress through the intricacies of denial was long and laborious. With patience and, for some, concealed frustration, group members used reason, arguments, personal examples, and stories to attempt to persuade Veronica that Zeke's actions were the result of Alzheimer's disease, and he could not help what he was doing. They tried to impress upon her that his brain was slowly dying. Eventually they were able to penetrate her stubborn, steadfast attachment to her denial. However, Veronica could not be pushed, prodded, or cajoled through this process. It was only when Veronica felt she had the inner resources to handle this challenge that she was able to come to grips with the fact that Zeke was indeed suffering from Alzheimer's disease and was not deliberately out to take vengeance on her. Then Veronica found that she could let go of her fear. Through education, validation, and the support of the group, she began to believe that she could do what needed to be done to take appropriate care of her husband of fifty-two years.

Elizabeth

Elizabeth was a retired high school teacher who was very involved in the city council and other political activities. She had rosy cheeks, short cropped gray hair, and was very spunky and vocal. In spite of the education she received in the group about the impact of Alzheimer's disease on the brain and how it affects behavior, Elizabeth continued to struggle with her denial of the consequences of this disease on her husband, Harvey, and their reasonable lifestyle. Once again in the group meeting, she bemoaned the fact that her husband "lied" all the time. She was furious, and there was an edge to her voice as she spoke to the group.

> Harvey lies all the time. The one thing I cannot tolerate is lying. He says he does not know where things are although he is the one who puts them away, and then he accuses me of hiding things and denies that he had anything to do with the lost item. It could be clothing, a book, money, anything. I just want him to tell the truth!

One of the group members, cognizant of Elizabeth's anger and identifying with her denial, empathetically stated, "You just don't want him to have this disease." Other members acknowledged her statement and showed their understanding; nodding in silence. Then Elizabeth said softly, "I wish my husband would just wake up tomorrow and be the way he always was."

Elizabeth, appreciative of the group's profound understanding, implored, "Please be patient with me. This is the hardest thing I've ever done."

Frank

Frank, a very strong, determined gentleman, was able to transcend his battle with denial and redirect his energy and passion toward more realistic and productive activities.

> Frank had sold his small manufacturing business back east and retired to Southern California with his wife, Olympia, so they would be close to their two daughters and their families. He was an energetic, "take charge" kind of guy, who had confidently controlled his business and had made the major family decisions for years. Early in his wife's illness, true to his char-

acter, he believed that he could, and without a doubt would, find a way to cure her. Thus, he aggressively began his quest. Frank sent for information from a multitude of sources and networked throughout the country with various Alzheimer's disease research groups. During one of my visits, he told me he was seriously considering moving them to Texas for a few years, as there was a potential cure being offered by a research group there. However, after further investigation, he decided their results were really not plausible enough to warrant such a major change. Instead he decided to enrole Olympia in an experimental drug study at the local university.

Six months later, when I arrived at Frank's apartment, he was furious. He had just found out that Olympia had probably been on a placebo in the research study. He had also exhausted all other resources. The reality that he was not going to find a cure, because one didn't exist, and that he was not capable of restoring his wife's health, seemed to demoralize him. However, as these strong feelings dissipated, he gave himself permission to stop chasing the fantasy. Also, after adamantly denying, during this time, that a support group could be helpful, he finally decided to attend one.

By my next visit, six months later, with the same gusto by which he lived his entire life, he had become a regular member of two groups, an active advocate for caregivers, and was helping them resolve some of their legal, financial, and health insurance problems. Frank lightheartedly added that he took his anger out on the golf course and responded to his wife with a patience of which he never thought himself capable.

Denial is a common, natural defense mechanism that we all use on occasion in order to cope with our surprise or shock about something that we are not ready to admit to or to handle. Denial is a necessary first step in many difficult events we may face in our lives: a loved one's death, a diagnosis of cancer, or other unexpected negative events. Because denial tends to keep one in a holding pattern, it becomes essential that we progress and move through it, so that we can once again feel empowered to move forward and get on with our lives.

Coincidentally, with Alzheimer's disease it may be the patient who, aware that something is not right, covers up and denies that anything is wrong or that help is needed. Sometimes caregivers collude in this denial, which can be risky and put your loved one in danger. A common example is allowing your spouse to continue driving the car because you both wish to continue believing that he or she is still a reliable, safe driver.

Therefore, in order to overcome denial, you must be patient with yourself and give yourself time to become educated about Alzheimer's disease and apply that knowledge to understanding and handling the abnormal behaviors in your spouse. The more you know, the harder it becomes to deny the facts. Once you acknowledge your loved one's diagnosis and assimilate your new learning, the more likely it is that you will begin to realistically deal with the behavior and other symptoms caused by Alzheimer's disease. Paradoxically, you will be freed from the grip of denial and will find the momentum that will allow you to move into action. Care management of your loved one can then be more appropriately and realistically planned according to the stage of the disease and your spouse's current needs.

RESENTMENT

Resentment usually increases as the disease progresses, since behaviors become more challenging and frustrating, and your life becomes more constricted. It is very difficult to understand the "why me" of this illness and not to resent the cards you have been dealt. As a spouse you may become embittered and resentful about the unwelcome but necessary role changes that Alzheimer's disease, by its very nature, demands from you as you are forced to put your life on hold. In addition, many caregivers relate to the thankless nature of caregiving, or to the reality that family and friends don't really understand how trapped you have become.

Let's examine the profundity of resentment for a moment. Why does this emotion develop the intensity that it does, and what can you do about it? It is common that Alzheimer's disease manifests itself with ambiguity, inconsistency, and inappropriate behaviors that also cause frustration and, at times, embarrassment. We need to factor into this the context of your relationship to your spouse at the onset of this unwanted crisis. If, historically, the relationship has been one that is disengaged, discordant, or unpleasant in any way, it's possible that your resentment has its roots in long-held feelings of anger and will therefore become even more intense. However, even if you have had a relatively good relationship, you can find yourself so entangled, so enmeshed with the patient and this unconquerable disease, that the churning of resentment is inevitable. At some level you have been ensnared in this glutinous trap of caregiving, and before you know it, you find the reliable, predictable patterns of your life have diminished. In attending to the chores and obligations and doing what needs to get done, you have had to put your own life on hold, often with never a thank-you or word of appreciation for all that you do. It's not unusual to find yourself feeling resentful toward the demands of taking care of your spouse and embittered and exasperated by the disease.

As we often mention in this book, you are constantly in the grip of several emotions, many experienced concurrently. For example, in an attempt to resolve some of the resentment, you may decide to step back from caregiving and reclaim parts of your life, but then find that when you do so, feelings of guilt begin to hover. In the middle of enjoying a time-out, a luncheon date or round of golf, for example, that old menace guilt appears and you begin to question yourself. "How could I be so selfish and irresponsible?" "What if something happens to my spouse when I'm not on task?" "What could I have been thinking?" You find yourself in a real Catch-22.

The same technique applied in coming to terms with resentment can be employed in dealing with other negative feelings. The first step is to understand and acknowledge the emotion as a normal feeling. Remind yourself that it's okay to feel this way. Then take action to move beyond it. With an emotion such as resentment, one helpful action involves taking time for yourself. In order to do a good job of nurturing yourself, it is important that you recognize that you're not selfish when you consciously choose to nourish and care for yourself. After all, the bottom line is, what will happen to your loved one if something happens to you? This question has been raised numerous times in our work with caregivers. It often has the effect of startling you enough so that you pause, take heed of warning signs, begin to cope differently and meet some of your own needs. Changing your thinking and behavior is vital to remaining both strong and healthy.

In assessing your own caregiving situation, you must reapportion and restructure your time, perhaps doing nothing extraordinary but revising and prioritizing your daily and weekly schedule. As the demands of caregiving change, it is critical to be flexible and readjust your plans from time to time. In this plan we strongly urge you to include a portion of fun or a relaxing time-out for yourself. Trade off and make peace with what really needs to be done and what can be done less often. Does Jane need a daily shower? What if you don't dust or make the bed today? Can you switch to paper plates for your sandwich at lunchtime? What about having pizza delivery or mobile waiter service once a week? Is it time to acquiesce to the fact that you can't do it all by yourself and engage extra help? It's very wise to know when to admit that you're not the only one who can give your spouse the care and attention that he or she needs. When you're able to step back and reassess your role, in order to regain structure and control and give yourself some respite from caregiving, your strong feelings of resentment will fade. You will discover as you prioritize that you do have choices. You don't have to put your life on hold, and you do not have to be responsible for every outcome. What a relief!

Anka

Anka's husband was sixty-two when he was diagnosed with Alzheimer's. She had worked as a legal secretary most of her life, but when Fritz retired from his accounting firm, Anka did the same. She and Fritz had traveled, entertained, and enjoyed going to the theater.

Over time, Anka could not get over her resentment that this illness had occurred and was changing her life dramatically. She felt that she really didn't deserve this. Everything that she had enjoyed was being taken away from her. Even though she persisted in taking haiku and line-dancing classes, Anka's feelings of resentment created such a black hole for her that nothing seemed to give her pleasure. At the urging of her social worker at the Alzheimer's Research Center, Anka joined a support group. There, she met two other women whose caregiving had given them a commonality. Since a major part of their resentment also revolved around loss of pleasurable activities, they decided that once a week they would do something fun together—go to a matinee and lunch, shop at a new mall, or play tourist in their own town. This was an excellent adaptive strategy.

In time Anka's resentment dissipated. While there was no answer for "why me," there was, in the evolution of Anka's new friendships, a possibility to rekindle old pleasures and invent new ones. In addition, the fun and camaraderie they experienced became the means that allowed Anka and her friends to dig out from under their negativity and have something to look forward to. Distracting herself from her resentful feelings by becoming involved in something fun, Anka found that she had more energy and could care for her husband more effectively.

Whereas Anka's resentment centered on her perceived losses in the quality and activities in her life, Bernice's was triggered by her husband's irrational behavior and her feeling that she had been robbed of a companion, and her husband of a decent retirement.

Bernice

Bernice worked as a part-time secretary, enjoyed homemaking and motherhood, and had been relatively content in her marriage to Eli. It had its normal ups and downs, but in the last few years, they seemed to grow closer and enjoyed each other's company very much.

Her husband had always been very physically active and energetic. Before retirement, he was a construction supervisor and had thoroughly enjoyed the outdoor nature of his work. He played soccer and tennis for years, until Alzheimer's disease interfered with his ability to compete. His behavior with Bernice had become uncontrollable and often aggressive. Bernice's resentment toward Eli and the illness grew. She felt that Alzheimer's disease had victimized them both.

She had joined the support group only a few months before she spoke up with a pained look on her face and in pure exasperation.

> I feel so many mixed emotions. Although Eli's behaviors continue to irk me, and sometimes even frighten me, when I look at this man, I realize how much he has been cheated. Cheated out of life! How much he is missing! He was fun loving and active, and now he's a victim. I hate this! I feel so sad about it that I cry a lot. God forgive me, but I wish he was more advanced in this disease so that he wouldn't be aware of what he has lost. He seems to be depressed, too. I resent the situation I've been placed in. I feel bitter and angry. I find myself frowning, pouting, and sulking. This is not me. I've lost myself, and I am really resentful about the whole thing.

This was the first time that Bernice had openly voiced such harsh feelings of resentment. However, it is through our emotions that we are compelled to take action, especially if we feel uncomfortable enough. Bernice, in airing her opinion and in receiving supportive comments and encouragement from the group over many months, was able to realize that she could gain control over some aspects her situation. She saw that her feelings of resentment were eating her alive and that she was losing energy to them. Her comrades in the group suggested that if she took this disease day by day, and tried not to compare today with the past or project into the future, she might find each day easier to cope with and live through. They also told her that they, too, had felt the same way initially. Some told Bernice that at times, they still felt resentful, but it wasn't as intense.

At a subsequent meeting, Bernice sat up straight in her chair and with an unwavering voice addressed the group.

> After many months of soul searching, I've finally realized that I can't deal with this situation as I have been. I love my husband and I'll take care of him as long as I can. I may get some in-home help and ask our children for some assistance. When I think of how good my life has been with Eli, my resentment seems self-serving. I'll make sure that he always has what he needs and accept that I may feel resentful at times. After all, I am a human being and these are normal feelings.

This understanding and change helped Bernice feel better and function with less disruptive emotionality. She also accepted help from her children and hired a caregiver to relieve her of some of her responsibilities. In doing so, she was able to look forward to some pleasurable activities and to nourish herself.

GUILT

It is very important to understand and analyze guilt; what it means, where it comes from, and how to come to terms with it. Other words that are synonymous with guilt are "culpability," "criminality," "lawlessness," "blame," "wrongful," "sinful" and "reprehensible." Be mindful of these words as you read the following commentary and conceptions regarding guilt.

Almost every caregiver with whom we've been in contact over many years, has been tormented by guilt. It has been the cause of much unnecessary anguish and despair. Note that guilt is not an emotion with which we are born. In order to understand the roots of guilt, it may be helpful if you would think back to your childhood. When did guilt begin to influence you? Perhaps you hit your brother or sister, spilled your milk, or took some cookies without permission. When found out, scolded, and disciplined, you may have believed that you were "bad," defective in some way, a disgrace, and with punishment, you felt condemned. Was the aberrant behavior evil, atrocious, rotten? We could guess that most of the time it wasn't. Through projections and indoctrinating views presented to us by parents, teachers, society, or religion at an early age, we form an interpretation of these "unacceptable" behaviors that develops into the idea that because we were the perpetrators of the behaviors we were "bad," without virtue or flawed. Because guilt is a learned response, we became apologetic and contrite in reaction to the belief that we had caused some harm. So began the birth of our conscience. With a conscience we can feel guilt, remorse, contrition, disappointment, and apologetic in ourselves. It is healthy to have a principled and moral code by which we live that doesn't allow us to deliberately and knowingly harm another or commit an immoral or illegal act.

With guilt, we suffer great emotional pain, especially when we believe that others disapprove of us or that we are bad. We feel guilty and accept that we deserve to be punished. When you are experiencing feelings of guilt, ask yourself, "What bad thing have I done?" Do you qualify as a bad person because you think, "I wish my spouse would leave and never come back?" What if you lost your temper and yelled at your spouse? Are you bad for doing that? Let's hope you can separate and see the difference between a negative thought or act and being a bad person. We all have limitations. Let's look realistically at the situation you're in. As a caregiver, you have in all probability been exerting extraordinary effort over time and are feeling depleted, physically ill, or just all done in. Look at the tasks you are performing in a twenty-four-hour day; tasks that are nerve-wracking, strenuous, exhausting, and seem to be never ending. As a longtime caregiver in the support group, Angela used to remind her fellow attendees that they were not leading a normal life and that these were not normal times. She would emphasize that a caregiver's days are fraught with ambiguity, inconsistency, and constant readaptation.

Often as a caregiver you put yourself in a catch-22 or no-win situation. When overworked and run-down, you may relent and get other help for your spouse so that you can take a break. However, even in making a healthy and rational decision by reassigning some of your daily burdens, you may feel guilty and let the power of that guilt undermine the rest and peace of mind you were seeking and truly deserve. When your coping abilities are compromised by your exhaustion, can you forgive yourself, love yourself, and let go of guilt? You are, after all, human and frail—a mere mortal.

Dr. Rudolf Dreikurs, in his teachings about the psychology of mankind, would often encourage his patients and his students to develop "the courage to be imperfect." Perfection can be found in nature in butterflies and flowers, perhaps, but as mortals we waste time striving for that unattainable goal. By acknowledging your imperfection, you can gain better control of the negative thoughts, feel less guilt, and move forward. Vanquish guilt and its accomplices: self-judgment and self-criticism. Accept who you are. Acknowledge that you're doing the best you can.

Evelyn

Although Evelyn mentioned, during my first visit with her, that she felt guilty about her husband having this illness, it wasn't until our second meeting that it became a more vexing issue. Evelyn and I were sitting at her dining room table during the interview when her husband, Stan, walked in. She fabricated an entire story for him in order to explain what I was doing

> there. I was a little surprised until she told me that she never discusses Alzheimer's with Stan and that she certainly does not want him to think that she is his caregiver. He has always denied that he has Alzheimer's. Therefore she creates any means necessary to cover for him and allow him this deception. Evelyn's guilt was twofold. She was feeling guilty not only because Stan had this illness, but also because she was constantly lying to him and colluding with him in this fantasy. Evelyn, in clarifying her stand, said she was so afraid that Stan would become terribly depressed if he ever acknowledged his illness. She believed that the longer she could protect Stan from this knowledge, the longer she could stave off any depression. Not being honest with Stan and going against her moral standard placed Evelyn in a catch-22 position. The discomfort heightened her guilt and also the self-loathing that was developing. Evelyn needed to be supported and educated about the impact of guilt and to look objectively at her behaviors and her thoughts. She had to reframe her view of herself.

Evelyn began to understand that lying out of benevolence, allowing Stan to retain his dignity, may have served a positive purpose larger than the "sin" of the lie itself, and she was able to come to terms with the exaggerated guilt and self-loathing.

Mannie

Mannie, who was ordinarily a delightful, jocular caregiver, often sharing a humorous story or a good laugh, became quite serious on the day he told the group of his feelings of guilt since he had placed his wife, Rachel, in day care. As he spoke, he bowed his head, and his usually playful persona disappeared.

> Rachel and I have always enjoyed each other's company, but I can't say that this is true these days. Her repetitive behav-

> iors, afternoon pacing, constant shadowing and questioning, had been driving me nuts. I turn around and boom, there she is right in my face. I've had to send her to day care a few days a week in spite of my vow to keep her at home. Boy! Do I feel guilty! I broke a promise, and I feel as if I've cast her away, forsaken her, let go of responsibility. Rachel seems to enjoy the days that she attends day care and comes home so tired she's easier to take care of. I know that she's in the right place. Yet, I feel so guilty about sending her out of the house! I decided to discuss my feelings of guilt with my rabbi. I'd like to tell you something that he told me, that might help you, as it seems to have changed my overwhelming struggle with guilt. He pointed out that the experience of guilt, while negative, actually allows us to carry out the appropriate task. My guilt came from feeling that I was really doing something for myself, being selfish, in putting Rachel in day care. So in feeling guilty I could punish my self enough to feel less selfish and continue with the good and practical decision to have Rachel in day care. It sounds convoluted but it actually makes sense.

We all have a desire to do good by our actions and therefore to feel satisfied about who we are. As caregivers, it is a sense that we have lived up to our obligations. When Mannie placed Rachel, he believed that he had not carried out his perceived and personally defined obligation to care for his wife. Instead, he had handed her care over to someone else. He abandoned her. Mannie placed Rachel in day care because he realized he needed a break, time to recoup. What he did is reasonable; however, he was afraid that it appeared that he was more concerned with his welfare than with the needs of his wife. This may sound familiar, as we have observed it time and again with our caregivers. But is it rational?

Can you also perceive how self-punitive guilt can be? In this sense, as caregivers, it seems that carrying guilt around is rather fruitless. Why add another burden to your shoulders? You are in a unique situation where certain actions are required in order for you to maintain your health and sense of well-being to the best of your ability. Feelings of guilt can be destructive and can interfere with your ability to make rational decisions. If Mannie's guilt were to continue, it would be important to seriously consider this feeling to be a symptom of depression or an expression of great sadness and grief. Suffice it to say, however, Mannie has been able to deal with his guilt in a healthy and positive way. He was able to set healthy boundaries in staying connected with his loved one, while letting go of the impossible, mistaken belief that he and only he could attend to all of her needs.

FEAR

In our close work with family caregivers, we have observed that feelings of apprehension and fear are universally present at some level. Caring for a loved one with Alzheimer's disease can easily cause you to begin to feel vulnerable and afraid. The most obvious case is if your patient becomes violent, although that happens in only a small percentage of Alzheimer's patients. However, other causes of fear, often less tangible, may abound. As a caregiver, you are trudging through unknown and unpredictable territory. Relationships change and can leave you feeling isolated and alone. You have inherited a tremendous and un-asked for responsibility. Decisions and their repercussions are often on your shoulders alone. The quality of your life has become fragile, and your security threatened. It is not uncommon for you to fear for your own mental competence. As you become busy and tired, your ability to retrieve a word, remember where you put something, or concentrate may seem impaired. You may worry that your children could inherit this illness. Your own health may decline. You may be encountering financial instability. You may fear that you are not going to be able to cope. It's important to note that all of these fears are legitimate in themselves, that is, they are possibilities based in reality. They are valid. It is important to distinguish a fearful situation from what is perhaps imagined and becomes inordinately feared in your psyche. You must act reasonably and often quickly to improve, eliminate, and defuse fearful situations. However, it is most important to keep perspective and not become overwhelmed or distraught by overexaggerated and unrealistic fears, so that you can continue to feel empowered and competent as a caregiver.

Although not a norm, dealing with a violent patient is traumatic, and effective action needs to be taken to protect yourself and others. We'd like to share with you Lily and Elizabeth's experiences.

Lily

It was always a pleasure to visit Lily, a beautiful, optimistic, genteel southern woman whose home was spotless, decorated with her Lladro collection and fresh flowers from her garden on every table. As her husband, Dick, became more paranoid in the middle stages of his illness, Lily became more and more fearful. His mild paranoia changed to verbal abuse and threats of violence. In their marriage, Dick had cherished Lily and held her in the highest esteem. Now he called her a whore and accused her of having an affair with Pete, their dear friend and neighbor next door. Lily cried as she told me how degraded she felt, even though she knew her husband didn't really know what he was saying. Furthermore, she was humiliated to tell Pete, their neighbor, that he must never come to help them anymore or even talk to her over the fence. Pete had been a supportive friend, and as Dick became less capable of caring for the yard or maintaining the house, he had graciously helped them. Dick also imagined that Lily was having an affair with the "man in the mirror." He didn't realize that it was his reflection that he was seeing. In fear that he would hit the man in the mirror and injure himself, she removed the mirrors where possible and covered the others over. Although he had never hit Lily, he had raised a hand to her on more than one occasion. Fearing for her safety, she was able to run out of the room and away from Dick. She exclaimed to me that she was tense and frightened most of the time.

I had urged Lily to talk to Dick's doctor about his aggression and paranoia, and explained that there are medications to temper these behaviors. Sensing that Lily was very vulnerable, I encouraged her to seek the help of a therapist for herself and attend a support group where she could learn how to deal with problem behaviors. As convincing as I thought I was, I left Lily's with a sense that she was still not ready to accept my recommendations, mired as she was in attending to Dick day to day.

When I visited Lily six months later, I was taken aback by the toll Dick's behavior had taken on her. She looked bedraggled. This incredibly optimistic, vibrant woman was hardly able to get through the daily chores. More importantly, she could not shake the feelings of fear, worthlessness, and degradation. At the insistence of her family, she told me that she had finally decided to see a therapist and had an appointment the next week. I was very relieved that Lily's family had interceded and hence she was taking an active step in caring for herself. She was at a breaking point.

On my subsequent visit, six months later, Lily seemed more like her old self again—full of optimism, energy, and hope. Fresh flowers were back on all of her tables. Her therapist had put her on an antidepressant for the time being and involved her in talk therapy. Dick's physician recommended that he be placed on a mild antipsychotic to treat his paranoid, aggressive, and agitated behaviors. He had also given her some steps she could take to disarm some of Dick's aggressive behaviors. His suggestions were that Lily should always approach Dick from the front, talking to him calmly and explaining slowly what she wants him to do, step by step; she could also avoid conflict by agreeing with Dick or distracting him; if he became agitated, she should back off and wait a while before asking him to attempt the same task.

As you see, it was not over a period of a few weeks but over two years from the time of the onset of Dick's aberrant behaviors to the time Lily took the positive steps toward their resolution. Lily had come close to her breaking point, not realizing the toll the cumulative effect of living each day with fear was having on her. It's so important to be aware of warning signs of your own fragility and to seek help as soon as possible.

Elizabeth

Elizabeth had attended the caregiver group for two years. She was petite, quite pragmatic, not easily shaken, and was coping quite well with her husband, Harvey's, erratic behavior. She always asked a lot of questions and was eager to learn as much as she could, in order to help herself cope successfully with her situation. Fear arose one day when her husband of fifty-six years struck her.

> My husband has become quite insecure. He constantly shadows me, wanting to be close. Last Thursday I stepped into the bedroom, and when I turned around there he was. I am not sure what triggered his response, but before I knew it, he struck me, causing me to fall backward onto the bed. He lunged at me, and in order to defend myself, I put my legs up and kicked him in the abdomen. It was a reflex reaction. Harvey fell back against the wall, making quite a thump. I was horrified at what I had done, and was also aware of how scared I was. Luckily, my son was in the house at the time, and hearing the scuffle, he rushed into the room. He gently led Harvey out of the room, giving me some time to regain my composure. As you might predict, a half hour later, Harvey had forgotten the entire incident. However, I remained pretty shaken for many hours.
>
> It's a week later and we now have Harvey on medication—Haloperidol. Thank God, he is much calmer. I find I'm still nervous, and I feel the stress in my body. I'm afraid that I may

unknowingly provoke him again. I've read and heard enough over the years to realize that this stage will pass, and that sets my mind somewhat at ease. I know to be wary, but I can't allow myself to hang onto unpleasant incidents for too long. I'm also grateful to my dear children, who are so loving and helpful.

A major fear that many caregivers have expressed is their concern about what will happen to their loved one if their own health were impaired in a way that would prevent them from caring for them.

Olivia

Shortly after Gerhard was diagnosed with Alzheimer's, Olivia had a mild stroke. Her recovery was quite good, but the stroke left her with some occasional dizziness and weakness in her right leg. Because of these impairments, she readily gave up her driver's license. Gerhard was still able to drive with Olivia giving directions, but her fears were twofold. She knew that as the Alzheimer's advanced, it would no longer be safe for Gerhard to be behind the wheel. Even then he lacked judgment, had no sense of geography, and his ability to react quickly to situations was already compromised. She also feared that she might have another stroke. The insecurity over their safety and mobility was frightening.

For many years after Gerhard's retirement from the Navy, where he served as a naval architect, he and Olivia lived in a comfortable condominium overlooking the bay near the Navy docks. Gerhard occupied much of his time watching the Navy ships and recreational vessels navigate the harbor. The Navy had been his life and had taken both of them to many exotic stations over his career.

Olivia hated the idea of taking all of this away from Gerhard, whose memory still seemed quite active about the Navy, the ships, and the sea. She realized however that they

> should move closer to their children, where their safety and day-to-day living would no longer be constantly alarming and worrisome. It was a very big decision to make without Gerhard's input, but she consulted with all of her children and came up with a solution. Olivia, wanting to maintain as much independence as possible for everyone's sake, moved with Gerhard to a retirement village for military officers only minutes from one of their daughters. No longer close to the sea and having left many close friends, Olivia was dispirited for awhile, but at last she was no longer frightened. Surprisingly to her, however, Gerhard really didn't seem to miss the ocean and actually got on quite well with the other retired military officers, who were even quite tolerant of his repetitive stories.

It is profoundly important that you make plans in advance of any possible crisis. It was during group one day that the participants were asked to give some thought to this predicament and to be prepared to share some ideas with each other the following week. The following is what some of the support group members suggested if something unforeseen were to happen to them.

Angela

> I'd often thought about what would happen to Joe in the event that I became ill, and it has really bothered me, especially since my two daughters are so far away. I came up with a plan and approached my friend and next-door neighbor, Maureen, who kindly consented to take care of Joe over a short period of time in an emergency and until my daughters can get back into this country. I have written up a detailed account of Joe's schedule: what time he rises, the assistance he needs, what he eats, when he takes his medications, and what his toileting habits are. As Joe regresses, of course, I will need to revise the list. Maureen also knows how to contact my girls so that they

could make plans to come home. I know how difficult this will be for both my neighbor and my children. As much as I loathe the idea of being dependent on them, I realized I have to swallow my pride so Joe will not suffer if I have an emergency.

Nate

After last week's meeting, I gathered my children together and we brainstormed in order to develop an emergency plan if my old ticker goes or something else befalls me. The interesting thing is that it was easier for me to talk about my possible demise than it was to think of my wife's. However, we all met with an attorney, who drew up a new will and trust. Flora and I had previously signed living wills and had picked out our gravesite, which she called "our last home." We knew what her last wishes were and what sort of memorial service she desired. We prepaid for plots and caskets and all the paraphernalia. You know those fees can become excessive over time.

But what about the possibilities that I would fall ill or even die before Flora? We needed to talk about who would take over the care of my wife, their mother. This was hard. There were tears, fears, and some denial and resistance to looking at this potentiality. We persevered. Although I would have preferred that Flora be cared for in the home of one of the girls, I realized how much strain, tension, and tumult this could cause, especially over a protracted amount of time, on them, their marriages, and their children.

We agreed that they would all meet Flora's doctor and we would scout around for a facility that seemed to be nurturing and attentive to patients who suffered from Alzheimer's. In the interim, if Flora was on a waiting list, two of my daughters said they would be responsible for Flora in their homes and would bring in professional help to care for her in their absence.

> We ended this meeting emotionally worn but deeply gratified and confident that we had achieved a plan that would be effective and had given us all peace of mind.

To many families, such a satisfying plan of action coming out of a family meeting may not be so readily accomplished. You may need the skills and resources of an experienced therapist and possibly an attorney familiar with elder law issues. Your local Alzheimer's Association is always a reliable resource for information and referrals. There are several questions you should be able to answer in devising your own plans for your spouse. Can you name a trusted person who would be immediately able to step in for you? Does that person know the details of your spouse's needs? Have you identified a care facility for your spouse if need be and made some initial arrangements with them? Have you drawn up the appropriate legal documents which include a living will and financial provisions for the care of your spouse? Does a significant family member or friend know where all of your important documents are kept and have access to them?

These questions may seem to be upsetting, unbearable, cold, and perhaps premature, but it is very important not to put off dealing with these issues, primarily for the security and protection of your spouse and also for your own—as well as your family's—peace of mind.

FRUSTRATION

The feeling of frustration, normal and common to many caregivers, is yet another difficult and complicated emotion that can have severe repercussions for both you and your Alzheimer's spouse. It can be a fleeting reaction that has a negative effect on your composure and sense of control or can intensify to the point of defying reason. Since it is related to anger, it can quickly burgeon into rage, leading you to become hotheaded and volatile. Once you understand its machinations, you can, over time and with perseverance, begin to be more moderate, self-contained, and levelheaded in your reactions. Remember, one of your challenging tasks as a caregiver is to accommodate and adjust to this disease in such a way that you adapt with benevolence and compassion for both yourself and your patient. Alzheimer's disease is frustrating, and it is also a transformational experience for caregivers—one in which you incrementally progress and alter your outlook and behaviors. Often this occurs outside of your conscious mind. Throughout this caregiving experience, you subtly begin to realize how adaptable you are and how you can engage untapped skills and inner resources that you didn't even know were in your possession.

Dare we list the events that could be responsible for your feeling frustrated? Let's identify some of the origins. They undoubtedly include your loved one's annoying and repetitious behaviors; monotonous, recurring questions; poor manners, wetting clothes and bedding; and forgetfulness, to name an obvious few. The difficulty in putting these frustrations in perspective is compounded by your own intense daily involvement with your patient and your own weariness.

How do you deal with your feelings of frustration? Recognizing frustration as a problem is the first step. What drives you bonkers? When do you become exasperated? When you are able to be aware of the triggers, try to pay attention to your thoughts. What are you saying to yourself when you feel so frustrated? Do you recognize any of these statements: "He's doing this to me," "She never listens," "I have to repeat myself over and over again"? Our emotions make us vulnerable, and we react spontaneously to the thoughts we have, although we are often unaware of their content. In circumstances of high stress and low tolerance, your emotions can become volatile and out of control. The good news is that we have power over our thoughts and can therefore effectively alter or modify them. For example, you could be thinking that you cannot answer another inane question your spouse asks. You've been doing it all day every day for weeks. You've had to clean up his mess around the toilet twice. You shopped for groceries with his "help." He refused to eat his dinner and now is following you from space to space, perseverating incessantly. He asks again, "What time is it?" Boom! You've had it. The worst negative thoughts are going through your mind—"I can't cope with this any longer!" "I wish he'd disappear!" "I'm helpless!" thus triggering strong negative emotions.

The important thing to do is to attempt to name the thoughts and emotions that arise. At first this will seem impossible to do at that moment. That's okay. Changing your reactions and discovering your thoughts takes time, patience, and practice. It will be easier when you are able to calm down and get some clarity. Then go back in your mind to the event and decipher what your thoughts were telling you. The emotion may be anger, resentment, hatred, or frustration, for example. The thought may be: "I want to punch him in the chops," "What have I done to deserve this?" or "I just can't go on." Can you discover both the hottest emotion and the hottest thought connected to that emotion? It is crucial for you to understand that it is the thought that creates the feeling. Your feelings are created by what you are thinking. Try to notice and identify what sensations you feel in your body as you relive that troubling event. Name the sensations that arise. Perhaps your heart beats faster or you develop a headache or tightness somewhere in your body.

Let's say you're thinking that you can't go on for another day and that you're feeling completely frustrated. Think about what would have to happen differently for you to go on for another day and another and another. You may even conclude, very logically, that it's time for respite, time to give yourself a physical and emotional time-out. How can you handle each of the behaviors in your spouse that triggers your frustration differently? For example, if he continually shadows you, could you sit him in front of the TV and put on a National Geographic video? What about giving him some papers to stack or coins to sort through? Perhaps when you have your spouse settled, you could take a time-out in your room to rest, and tell him you'll be back when the timer goes off. As you turn your thoughts to positive alternatives, how are you feeling? What has happened to the frustration? What has happened to the tension in your neck? Hopefully you're feeling less frustrated, more competent, in control, and generally better about yourself.

It also may help to unload and discuss your frustrated feelings and negative thoughts with someone who will empathize and support your sentiments. Often, two heads are better than one. The two of you may be able to come up with several rational solutions to solve your problem. A therapist can help you deal with your irrational and sabotaging beliefs and guide you to more rational and functional beliefs that will allow you to gain skills and confidence in yourself.

In order to regain your equanimity, you could take a walk or soak in a tub, or have a cup of coffee or tea. Perhaps you could meditate, be lost in thought, and breathe consciously—long, slow, deep breaths. Focus only on your breathing for five or ten minutes. This will help you to regain your composure and balance and clear your mind. When more composed, you should be able to better envision an alternate approach to adopt in alleviating the frustrating behavior you confront.

Sylvia

A strong-willed and spirited caregiver, Sylvia had coped well with her husband, Phil's, irrational behaviors. She had two outlets that seemed to bring her a sense of well-being: Painting and meditating. When painting, she was completely immersed in that process and could let go of all other outside concerns. Meditation, practiced for thousands of years as a tool to quiet the mind and restore equilibrium, accomplished for Sylvia a similar goal. Surprisingly, one day, she came to the group meeting in tears. Her lips were tight and her face contorted as she reported her story with a loud, strident tone in her voice:

> I'm so frustrated with Phil these days, I could scream, and I do scream at him. I know I shouldn't, but it's getting bad. He disappears for hours. I drive around our entire complex looking for him, and when I haven't found him after a half hour or so, I finally give up. Thanks goodness the area is gated. But I get so frightened. I pray that a guardian angel takes care of him and brings him home safely. What else can I do? When he's in the house with me, I can't get anything done, and he undoes whatever I try to accomplish. His repetitious behavior is maddening. His inability to carry

> on a decent conversation leaves me frustrated and lonely. He eats too fast. Oh, I could go on and on. I'm at my wit's end. It's become impossible to paint or meditate, which would be so helpful in calming my mind. By the time he goes to bed, I'm emotionally and physically exhausted.

Her fellow comrades in the group, most of whom have had similar experiences, acknowledged Sylvia's palpable frustration. They understood very well. Some suggested that she have Phil attend day care for a day or two a week. Others suggested that she find something beneficial for both of them, like going for a drive along the water or taking a walk through the plaza. The caregivers' empathetic responses, along with their recommendations, helped Sylvia calm down. She realized that she did have some control, and she could make different choices that would help her to feel competent. After a bit, she said that she would think about sending Phil to day care. This would allow her to get back to her painting and meditation and just give her optional time. She acknowledged that she and Phil could still enjoy a drive or walks together and recalled how much they used to enjoy exploring the Southern California beaches.

When you're in the midst of frustration, it's so hard to step back and consider alternative ways of handling the difficult scenario with which you are confronted.

Carolyn

Being frustrated actually compelled Carolyn into some very clever and creative thinking. Her husband had become very restless at night. This scenario continued for months, and Carolyn ended up exhausted and feeling desperate.

> John was up at night continually. Night after night he'd suddenly get up and out of bed and begin to march. He was in the army years ago, you know. I tried to persuade him to get back

into bed. I'd show him the darkness outside and reason with him, telling him it was nighttime—sleepy time. I invited him to join me in bed. I tried everything.

Out of sheer desperation the other night, I had a grand idea. I decided to become part of his reality. To be where he really was at that time. So, I asked him what he was doing, how come he was marching and marching. He said that they marched him all of the time. He was annoyed. He asked me what they thought he could do, after all he's a man. How long could he hold out? I told John that he could simply stop and go to bed. Whereupon he emphatically stated that his commanding officer would not allow him to do that. So now I understood where he was, and without my knowing any military terms, I just shouted out, "Mr. Krantz, this is your commanding officer, Sergeant Patton. I am here to inform you that this is bed patrol and I am commanding you to return to bed immediately and get to sleep.

Well, I'll be darned if John didn't turn to me, salute, and quickly stumble into bed. He slept like a baby until morning. This has worked now for the last five nights.

Carolyn burst out laughing at this point and her friends in the group joined in. She had unwittingly demonstrated a key component to being a wise caregiver—rather than trying to deal with the patient reasonably and rationally, she joined him in his reality and connected with him where he was. Changing her focus and finding healthy alternatives saved the day, or, to be more accurate, the night, for Carolyn.

Nate

In this next vignette, although his wife's paranoid and delusional accusations frustrated Nate, he was able to find humor in what he often called the craziness of this whole disease.

A spunky eighty-year-old retired family practitioner, Nate thought caregiving would be second nature to him. However, he found himself continually struggling to be a good caregiver to his wife, Flora. When she became fixated on the imagined relationship between him and the home healthcare provider, who came to the house daily, his frustration became overwhelming.

> Sara had been hired as a daytime companion for my wife, so that I could get out on my own a few times a week. She seemed to be taking good care of Flora and even fixed a light dinner for us before she left for the day. Although I felt guilty at times, I was content to leave Flora in Sara's competent hands. I trusted her, and Flora seemed to get on well with her. After three weeks, out of the blue, Flora insisted that Sara be fired, saying that she was no good, she didn't like her. My guess was that she thought we were having an affair, but she couldn't really voice those fears. She had done the same thing with the two previous gals I had hired. Talk about feeling frustrated. I wanted to scream—yet another confounding obstruction thrown at me. I was bitterly disappointed and had finally acquiesced to Flora's demands to fire Sara, in order to keep the peace. Flora just wouldn't get off it. This time, even after I had fired Sara, Flora's paranoid and delusional behavior continued. Every time I was on the phone or leaving the house, Flora would become incensed and accuse me of continuing to be in touch with Sara. She would ruminate for hours and harass me about "that woman." No amount of reassurance dispelled her paranoia. I would hug her, tell her how much I loved her, and offer to let her speak on the phone so she would know that the person with whom I was conversing was not Sara. I desperately pulled out all the tricks—alas, to no avail.
>
> This maddening conduct went on for several months. It was really getting to me, and I felt this could be my undoing. Then last week Mannie and I came up with this crazy idea that we thought just might work. I felt as if we were back in college plotting some elaborate caper. Together we conspired that

> Mannie would call me with the news that Sara had died in an accident, and I would make sure that Flora was within earshot of the conversation. Well, the next day Mannie called. Knowing my wife could hear me; I exclaimed loudly, "Oh, no, are you sure? Sara died in an accident? How tragic." Then I hung up, turned to Flora, and told her the news. She shook her head, muttering how sad that was, and left the room. I felt a rush of jubilant relief. "Yes," I said to myself, "it's finally over." My celebratory sense of relief, however, was short-lived. Within ten minutes Flora returned to the room and said to me, "You don't think I believe that ridiculous story, do you?" I was dumbfounded.

Nate's story captivated the group, who had empathetically suffered with him through the first part of the story. But they couldn't help joining him and Mannie in fits of laughter by its end. Some applauded, tears streaming down their faces. Suffice it to say, Nate's wife, some months later, forgot about Sara. His story of Sara and his and Mannie's failed plot, devised out of desperation and foiled by Alzheimer's, lived on in the group and bore repeating from time to time with a great deal of chiding and good humor.

CHAPTER 9

Tears of Laughter: the Importance of Humor

Nate's story of frustration is the perfect segue into discussing the importance of a sense of humor and laughter in dealing with this grave illness.

Global peacemaker and author Norman Cousins, in his book *Anatomy of an Illness*, published over twenty years ago, is credited with having written the universal, scientific treatise on the effect of laughter and humor in healing the mind, body, and spirit. He literally laughed his way out of a disease that doctors were convinced was incurable. Cousins's research indicates "negative emotions produce negative chemical changes in the body." He wondered if it was "possible that love, faith, laughter and confidence . . . would have therapeutic value." We have provided information to you regarding negative emotions and thoughts and how you can be affected by them, behaviorally, physiologically, and spiritually and also suggested ways in which to deal with your thoughts and feelings. We hope this section on the benefits of laughter and humor will allow you to make yet another choice that has the potential to be a positive influence on you and your health. Discover the delights of humor, and take advantage of this very valuable healing tool. Even with your difficult challenges you can believe that it's still possible to laugh. That humor can put things in perspective.

Just as we've suggested that you have the power to change your thoughts and that they are under your control, so, too, is the way you view some instances that emerge in your daily activities as you tend to your loved one. Some of you may wonder how anything could be funny in your daily interactions with an Alzheimer's patient. However, lightening up, enjoying a hearty chuckle or deep belly laugh about something that occurred in your caregiving is really important. Remember that you are not laughing at your loved one, rather you're discovering levity within the situation brought about by the disease. There have been numerous times when members of the group have laughed heartily at a situation described by the caregiver that just happened to be very, very funny. It's that simple.

Jane

Jane giggled as she shared the following story with the group members.

> In the late-early stage of Alzheimer's, Mac and I began to have difficulty with our sexual relationship. It was, of course, sometimes embarrassing and frustrating. His memory would fade in and out so quickly. He would approach me in a loving but clumsy manner, maybe giving me a smooch or trying to figure out what part of me to touch. His little buddy would be hard, and I knew he wanted to have sex. I would think, "Uh, oh," but would nonetheless consent. Invariably, once we were in the bedroom, he would forget his invitation and, you know, er, lose it. However, sometimes a while later he would recall his suggestion but distort what had really taken place. He actually called our children on more than one occasion to tell them that their mother was not giving him any.

Fay

Fay never lost her sense of humor throughout Harry's Alzheimer's. Harry was a retired military officer who was heavyset, stubborn, and as a patient would often become oppositional. At the first signs of incontinence, Fay knew that she could no longer handle him and placed him in a nursing facility that had an Alzheimer's unit. She described an incident that occurred during her visit with him earlier in the day.

> I was walking down the hall with my Harry, holding his hand affectionately as always. Halfway to his room, I let go and stopped to talk to the nurse about Harry's diet. Less than a minute later, I turned around to rejoin him and he was walking down the hall, holding hands with a complete stranger. He hadn't missed a beat. That's my Harry.

Laughter influences us subconsciously. When you laugh you find yourself in a positive state of mind. Laughter is refreshing and increases your sense of well-being. Research on the benefits of laughter has demonstrated that it affects your immune system positively and reduces stress quantitatively.

THE POWER OF LAUGHTER

Laughter helps us lighten up so that we can cope better. When you're laughing, your whole perspective changes. We have noticed with many caregivers that even when scary or serious situations arise, they are able to adapt by using humor as a coping strategy, which paradoxically enables them to become less tense or angry and therefore deal with whatever transpired more effectively. You simply cannot hold on to negativity and experience positive thoughts and feelings at the same time. When we allow ourselves to laugh, we are choosing to make light of the incongruities of life. Believe it or not, this empowers us. I recall Bill Cosby stating, "if you can laugh at it, you can survive it." How true.

Bella

> In the middle of my visit with Bella, Sol was becoming very impatient and had asked many times, "Are we going to the store yet?" Of course Bella was sorry she had told him in advance that that's what they were going to do. Finally, she said, "Sol, why don't you get dressed and then we'll go." About forty-five minutes, later Sol came into the living room. "Let's go!" he demanded. Bella and I looked up and there was Sol in a dress shirt and jacket with sweatpants and over them a pair of white boxer shorts emblazoned with big red and blue stars. He was such a sight! Bella and I laughed even though she knew she would have to start all over again with helping him dress before they went out. Philosophically, she said to me, "At least it gave us another forty-five minutes together." Gently and patiently she led Sol away, cajoling and teasing him as they headed toward the bedroom.

Laughter and playfulness increase our compassion for others and ourselves. Laughter helps us to cope better. It acts as a distraction. A good laugh helps us to put things in perspective. We have found that so many caregivers with whom we have worked gain strength in mirth. Sometimes in sharing a challenging event with the group, all of a sudden the humor of it can surface during the telling of it, changing the focus for a moment from troublesome to hilarious, from somber to silly. So many times caregivers have giggled or laughed out loud and infected others with jocundity and joviality in reliving an amusing moment. Try it. We highly recommend this coping strategy.

CHAPTER 10

The Mars and Venus of Adapting to Change: Gender Differences

As Alzheimer's disease progresses, you continue to adapt to the daily tasks of your caregiving situation, becoming increasingly resilient and tolerant of your spouse's unpredictable behavior. Gaining mastery and beginning to feel competent in their new role, most caregivers not only meet this unwelcome venture into precarious territory with success, but are also transformed by this experience.

There are several components necessary for this transformation to take place. At the outset, caregivers who are realistic, resilient, and optimistic are at an advantage. These characteristics enable the caregiver to recapture a sense of control, which is the very essence of coping successfully with Alzheimer's disease.

For many caregivers, it is the passage of time that allows them to ease into an adaptive mode. It's almost like navigating constantly forward through a dark tunnel until eventually one sees a glimmer of light at the other side. This is when you begin to nod silently as you look back at the distance traveled and, with hope rising, move onward, acknowledging your sense of mastery.

Transformation is facilitated in a milieu, such as a support group, where as caregivers you are allowed to express and reveal your most intimate feelings and thoughts. In such a nonjudgmental environment, you will encounter a sense of belonging and feel supported, understood, and encouraged. It's essential that you reach out to friends, family, church or synagogue, and/or therapist and also to a support group, where there is the unique experience in commonality. The fundamental issue for the caregiver is that you feel validated and reassured in the decisions you make.

Emotions, including anger, resentment, embarrassment, fear, guilt, and depression, are universal, and both male and female caregivers experience the gamut of sentiments. Given the same problems of adapting to the role of caregiver, however, the two sexes seem to adjust somewhat differently.

The question posed to the group at one meeting was: "How does Alzheimer's disease affect you and how did you adjust, or come to terms with this illness?" In general, women agreed that they tended to automatically assume the role of caretaker/nurturer, as it was an extension of the familiar role they had always had. Adding new tasks with which they were unacquainted and unskilled, such as dealing with finances or maintaining the car, shook their self-confidence and sometimes overwhelmed them. Men, on the other hand, believed that they were the providers, protectors, and were more pragmatic, feeling a strong need to fix the problems around the illness before they could begin to address the challenge of becoming caretaker/nurturer.

Another difference we discovered was that women generally form supportive networks to help them cope, while men often prefer to battle their situation alone. Often in the home visits for the study, when the possibility of attending a support group was recommended, the male caregivers would shun the suggestion and defend against it, whereas women were often willing to at least give it a try. Additionally, in most support groups, there is a higher ratio of women to men in attendance.

The following stories will help you to see how some male and female caregivers have perceived their situations.

Nate

The way I see it, as men, we want to do everything in our power to protect our spouse. I actually think it's more primal than that; I believe we are expected to be the protectors. Second, men want to fix, to do, to make something happen—we must have a solution. Consequently, it has been hard on my male ego to be stymied and not find answers and feel I'm failing in my role as the protector. In fact, it's taken me many grueling, soul-searching months to finally find the courage and common sense to give up this mission to cure Flora and adapt to the task of actually taking care of her. Who would ever have predicted that I would be cooking, doing the laundry, and even helping my wife to dress and undress? I never thought I could attend to her bathroom needs either. Do you remember my asking you ladies about the right way to wipe Flora after she urinated? Much to my surprise, I've discovered that I do have the ability to nurture and care for my wife. That makes me feel good. I started out as if superior to this illness in some way and was rather arrogant. I was also convinced that I could find a cure. I am justifiably humbled.

Bill

I agree with Nate and would like to add to what he said. With Alzheimer's disease, the diagnosis is so tenuous. Even if you go through the comprehensive testing with your spouse, the resulting diagnosis is possible/probable Alzheimer's disease—too much uncertainty for me. I had to question what this was all about, and I felt driven to find out as much as I could and to obtain some concrete answers. I took my Hazel to numerous specialists, hoping for a definitive diagnosis. I was feeling very insecure with this ambiguity. As an attorney, I could always come up with a successful solution to so many messes that my clients would get into. Researching Alzheimer's disease was so frustrating because there was no satisfactory outcome. Bottom line, right now there is no cure. Now, as I look back, I realize that because of who I am, I wouldn't have felt satisfied with my performance if I had not first gone through the process of researching and seeking answers and solutions. Having done so, I was then ready to accept the vagaries of Alzheimer's disease and to deal with my wife's decline to the best of my ability.

I must tell you that in all honesty I felt like a failure for a long time. I saw myself as a quitter. Then I became scared. I didn't know how or where to begin to help Hazel. When she needed assistance around the house, I was like a bull in a china shop. When I started cooking or grocery shopping I felt disoriented, like a mouse in a maze. Hazel had sailed through these chores in addition to taking care of our children, and I never appreciated how organized and adept she was. Until now, I hadn't shared this information about my struggles with anyone. I feel relieved to have unburdened myself. Thanks for listening.

Thelma

During my six-month visit with Thelma, she explained how initially unwilling and unsure she was in assuming her husband's role. However, adapting to new tasks out of necessity had changed her life.

It was only after Gray bounced a couple of checks that I began my new "career" as CFO of our household. Until then, and for the last forty years, I hadn't even been a co-signee on any banking accounts. I was worried sick and had no confidence in my ability to take over the finances, which included our personal stocks, retirement account, and taxes. We'd been talking for years about updating our will and trust but never got to that either. Unfortunately, Gray does not have a living will and at that time I didn't even have Durable Power of Attorney. In searching for reasons to feel optimistic, all I could think of was that I was always pretty good in math in high school. Don't laugh! You have to start somewhere. I soon found that the checkbook was easy. The children were encouraging and helped me outline what steps I needed to take. For the first time in our marriage, I talked to our accountant, lawyer, and financial advisor. I took my time and asked many questions and actually understood most of what they were talking about.

Slowly, with their help, I got everything in good order. It was a real sense of accomplishment and quite a relief. Much to my amazement, the money management fascinated me. Through an adult education program, I took a class on retirement investments and then a class on the stock market. I surprised myself with my competence and how much fun I was having. Now I meet regularly with our broker to discuss our portfolio and actually make joint decisions on my purchases.

For the first sixty-five years of my life, my role as a female was defined for me by societal expectations. My goal was to marry well and to be a good homemaker and mother. That experience has been invaluable in becoming a nurturing, patient, and competent caregiver to Gray. It has been an astounding leap for me to traverse that indelible gender line and function competently in what was defined in my generation as strictly a male domain.

Yvette

Like Thelma, Yvette's challenge in adjusting to and coping with Richard's declining abilities required a change of giant proportions for her.

> Ours was a traditional marriage from the get go. Before Alzheimer's, our roles were pretty clearly defined. I shopped for groceries, cooked, cleaned, and cared for the children. Richard was the breadwinner. I always relied on him to maintain the house, do repairs and light carpentry. Now he can't tell the difference between a pair of pliers and a hammer and also doesn't know what to do with either of them. I remember when Richard first began to show signs of dementia; he was really clumsy and inefficient in doing even simple jobs. He would forget to replace screws, or take things apart and never put them together again. When I'd remind him to finish something, he'd mutter some excuse and change the subject, leaving me frustrated and angry with him. Yet, I balked at the thought of entering his turf. Eventually, when reality hit and I accepted that Richard was no longer competent as the man of the house, and the house seemed to be slowly falling apart around me, I nervously began to take on this unfamiliar "masculine" role.
>
> Now I know how to fix leaky toilets, dripping pipes, set automatic timers for the garden, and even take care of our finances. I'm so proud of myself. To think I always believed this was men's work. It's been a challenge, and I'm very grateful to the men at the hardware store and my neighbors, who patiently walked me through the steps in home repair. At first I was embarrassed to tell my girlfriends what I was doing, but now I'm as pleased as punch with how handy I've become, and I want everyone to know.

What helped Yvette was her willingness to be flexible and to take a risk, as well as her belief that an "old dog can learn new tricks." The group cheered for her and one of the men lightheartedly asked her what she charged to repair a leaky faucet. The respect from the group was obvious and Yvette beamed.

Frank

Frank's struggles with his additional roles were more challenging than he had anticipated, except in the kitchen, where he felt right at home. His early passion for food and cooking became therapeutic when he was forced by his wife's illness to remain at home more and give up other outlets like golf and working out in the gym in order to maintain his peace of mind.

> I grew up in an Italian family and learned to cook in my grandmother's kitchen. I'd stand on a stool with her apron tucked up and wrapped around me. She taught me how to pare and dice and how to knead the noodle dough to the right consistency of moisture and softness. I preferred cutting ravioli to shaping the gnocchi but became pretty good at both, even though I'd be covered in flour from head to toe by the end. I remember the smells of garlic sautéing in olive oil and basil picked fresh from the garden. As an adult, however, the only time I cooked was on summer vacations in our house on the Jersey shore.
>
> When Olympia became ill, I started cooking simple recipes, but before long I was trying every marinara sauce I could find to decide which was closest to Grandma's. She never used a recipe. I did the same experimentation with baklava, which my wife's family always made. The neighbors in the apartment building were the grateful recipients of my cooking fugue, and I ended up regularly feeding a couple, who were battling the effects of AIDS.

It was my remembrance of the warmth and love that came out of my grandmother's kitchen that transformed my sanity. When I was cooking I felt peaceful and grounded.

Another contrast in acclimating to their new role as caregivers is that women generally are more comfortable forming supportive networks, whereas men tend to battle things out on their own. Proportionately, usually more women are open to joining support groups, and men often need to be prodded and cajoled.

Leonard

When Leonard joined the caregiver's group at the urging of his children, his wife, Rene, was well into the middle stages of Alzheimer's disease and caregiving had become pretty difficult. Initially, one of his children had attended the group with him, easing him into this situation. He discovered that what really helped him was hearing from the other men in the group, who welcomed him and shared their experiences of caring for their wives. To his surprise he found their stories very similar to his own, and they validated what he was feeling and going through. In the course of time Len began to feel a sense of pride and belonging and also began to openly share his challenges and triumphs.

As an aside, shortly after becoming a regular at the support group, Leonard would bring in a plate of homemade treats. Each week he would alternate; one week he would bring homemade blueberry muffins and the following week his brownies. Over time the group began to depend on him for his yummy munchies, and on one occasion when he came empty-handed they all playfully scolded him.

It was at one of the meetings that Len reflected on his evolution in facing the role and status changes as Rene's husband and caregiver.

Rene and I have had a very good marriage. It will be forty-nine years next month. All this time we kept the traditional female and male roles and that worked very well for us. Then boom, almost out of the blue, she began to change, leaving me confused, afraid, and lonely. I was losing not only my spouse, but also my friend, confidante, and longtime companion. Boy, those early years were rough, but I was determined that I could tough it out alone. I was resolute. However, I began to feel pretty run-down, so I went to the doc thinking he could give me some vitamins or a shot of something. He immediately recognized the exhaustion and also the isolation and a lot of other feelings churning inside of me. He insisted on my joining a support group, and when I told my daughter, she dragged me here. I came quite reluctantly, determined that this would be a onetime visit.

I am grateful. It was a big thing for me to learn to share the intimate and private details of our relationship and some of the embarrassing goings on in our household. But you really understood. Nothing seemed to surprise you. Besides that, you offered me support and advice on taking care of my wife and myself. You encouraged me especially to try things I've never tried before. In fact, some of you guys even challenged me.

I've become pretty adept and even creative in handling Rene's daily needs. Don't laugh at me when I tell you what I've learned to do for her. In the beginning I used to take her to the hairdresser once a week, but that soon became a hassle because Rene was uncooperative. I decided I would try to fix her hair myself. Now, I shampoo her hair, roll it up, and even tint it every four weeks. Rene always took pride in her appearance, and I am determined to preserve her dignity. She was a classy dresser, too. When I help her dress, I choose an outfit that is color coordinated, usually in her favorite hues of blue or rose. She looks like a doll.

Strange thing is that I find the more I am willing to do for her, the closer I feel to her. I grieve for what was, don't get me wrong. After all, she devoted her life to caring for me.

CHAPTER 11

The Lonely Bed: Adapting to Profound Loss of Intimacy

As Alzheimer's disease progresses, both caregiver and patient experience the bittersweet loss of appropriate physical intimacy and companionship. As Bonnie Genevay, gerontologist and bereavement consultant explains, "An elder's physical, mental, emotional, psychological, and spiritual heath all depend to some extent on the level of intimacy in their lives. Expressions of intimacy can invigorate older people and give them a sense of connection to their world." In older adult relationships, the response and intervals between sexual activity may slow down, but we acknowledge its importance even at a different intensity. The loss of the caressing touch, hugs and kisses, as well as intercourse is immeasurably disheartening for many caregivers and their spouses. When Alzheimer's is present, this important facet of the relationship eventually becomes a treasured, faded memory. Many caregivers reluctantly come to terms with this void in their lives as they express lack of fulfillment and profound grief over this significant loss.

However, even though sexuality and intimacy remain important components in the marital relationship, they are rarely openly discussed. Many caregivers will indirectly allude to this loss by declaring that they miss being hugged or that their spouse no longer finds them attractive. It is more often in private that some caregivers unburden themselves and reveal that sexual expression in the relationship has diminished completely and that they still long to be able to make love with their partner. When you become a caregiver, the basic human pleasure of being caressed, kissed, or in any way physically passionate does not just disappear, but for reasons specific to the fact that your spouse has Alzheimer's disease, the desire has been despoiled. There are many reasons why sexuality becomes a problem. One has to do with your changed role. Your customary status of wife or husband has evolved into that of parent or nurse as you nurture and tend to the needs of your demented spouse. It's as if you're now attending to a dependent child, as you did when your own children were young. Along with this, your afflicted spouse may no longer desire a sexual relationship, or may make inappropriate, displeasing sexual overtures. He may even suggest a rendezvous in the bedroom, only to forget or become distracted once in the room, causing frustration as well as an unfulfilled experience for you. Important as well, is that your spouse can no longer connect with your feelings or needs, such as knowing when you might want a hug or are in need of being comforted.

For many, lovemaking offers comfort and security and gives a sense of belonging within a relationship. Therefore, when this significant feature of affiliation disappears, you can and do feel neglected, rejected, and dissatisfied, which then can affect your disposition. Longing, loneliness, and depression are very common experiences for the caregiver, who, in addition to feeling abandoned by friends and family, now also feels estranged from his or her marital partner.

UNDERSTANDING SEXUAL BEHAVIOR IN ALZHEIMER'S

In some cases, the patient may still demonstrate an interest in sexual expression with his or her spouse. Some caregivers may oblige and engage in intercourse. However, many caregivers report that it was more like a "duty" than a satisfying experience, because the gratification and pleasure of foreplay and caressing and the emotionality were missing or clumsy and perfunctory. Thus, coitus becomes far from satisfying. Other caregivers have expressed with distaste how abhorrent and aversive the experience has become, and that they find they actually recoil from advances.

It is important to note that inappropriate sexual conduct is not very common in Alzheimer's patients. Engaging in this behavior is due to the disordered brain and not carried out to deliberately cause embarrassment. You know that when your spouse was well, such gestures or actions would never have been a part of his characteristic behavior. However, if your spouse does engage in publicly disturbing behaviors such as masturbation, fondling, or exposing himself, or makes inappropriate, aggressive advances toward you at home, it is crucial to know what to do about it. The best way to respond is quietly and gently. At home, if your spouse begins to fondle himself, lead him into the bedroom and onto the bed, so that if he wishes, he can continue in private. This behavior may feel satisfying or pleasing to your spouse.

In the case of unwanted behaviors, distraction is an acceptable alternative. If that approach is ineffective or the problem is more onerous or public, you may consider asking the doctor for a mild sedative for the patient until this phase passes, and it will. With one of the caregivers, her spouse would walk up to any female—a nurse, a store clerk—and aggressively try to pinch, hug, or kiss her, which was obviously mortifying for everyone but her husband. He was put on a medication that calmed his instinctual drive, and the problem dissolved instantaneously.

Angela

Angela had often spoken of the blow she felt over the loss of sex and companionship she had enjoyed with her husband of almost fifty-five years. One afternoon she shared the following touching story with the support group.

> Joe was such a loving man. He was always reaching for my hand or putting his arms around me. I felt so feminine and desirable. I long for his caring embrace and gentle touch. Touching was so important to us. I know that intercourse is gone forever. It seems that the more this disease devours his brain, the more physically distant we become. It's miserable. I have wrestled with this estrangement for a long time, and recently I had an idea that came out of an impulse to comfort him. Joe was standing in the hallway looking confused and forlorn, and my heart went out to him. I said to him as gently as I could, "Joe, I think you need a hug." He smiled and nodded back. We held each other in the hallway for a long time. Gosh, it felt so warm and wonderful. I finally got it. I've realized that Joe is no longer able to approach me, so I have to make the first move. We have continued to hug every day, and so far it's been very gratifying to both of us.

For the Caregiver Study, one of the questions we asked the caregivers was, "Do you still have intimacy with your spouse?" I usually would get a little nervous laughter as a response, and I would reply, "Is that a yes or a no?" Sometimes, however, it would give an opening to a caregiver who was having a great deal of difficulty with this loss. No one else usually ever asks that question. For Al, a dashing man in his early seventies, it was a real catharsis as he responded.

Al

> Wow, Mary! You don't leave a stone unturned. You know, I've had a really hard time with this. Part of the success and happiness in our long and happy marriage was that for all those years we had a very active and healthy sexual relationship. I miss it, Mary, and I don't know what to do about it. I agonize about the guilt I have for still wanting sex with Peg. I just feel that I would be taking advantage of her if I attempted anything. I lie next to her in bed at night and long for her closeness. Gee, I feel embarrassed telling you this. I miss so many things in the marriage, but I seem to come up with a practical solution for them. But this one has me stymied.

We talked about those feelings of arousal being quite normal and that it was understandable that the loss was very great for him. Also, I again encouraged him to attend a support group, where he would realize that he was not the only caregiver who was experiencing these feelings and would therefore no longer think of himself as a pariah.

Particularly for Al and his generation, discussing sexual intimacy, masturbation, and orgasm is difficult. However, with the trust of the support group, these subjects are safe. Al may have felt more validated by stories that came from group members, who were open and willing to share their feelings about this loss, as the next two vignettes illustrate.

Mannie

> We ought to admit it. We are no longer married in the traditional sense. We caregivers are more like married widows and widowers. It's an unusual situation. I never expected our marriage would end this way. I have been thinking back to the initial stages of this blasted disease and trying to make sense of all the crazy behaviors that are caused by it. At first I didn't

realize that Rachel was ill, although I did notice peculiar changes in her. As I thought about it more, I suddenly realized that it was fairly soon after her diagnosis that she stopped hugging me. When I began to acknowledge that these changes were due to Alzheimer's disease, I felt less rejected.

Still, my sexual needs go unsatisfied. It's a dilemma for me, and sometimes I think that I should find a companion. I can't believe I'm confessing this to you. I feel like a traitor. Nevertheless, at this point, I cope by being more loving to Rachel, and seeing how this helps her, is very rewarding for me. I find that at times, I don't want sex; I just want to hold her and be held. So I hold Rachel, stroke her hair and cheek or rub her back, and she seems to enjoy this as much as I do. I need affection and think that maybe Rachel needs it even more. The consequence of these tender moments is different each time. Sometimes we smile and look into each other's eyes, sometimes we're tearful, and other times we might squeeze just a little harder. This helps me go on with my own life and look at what I can still preserve, rather than pitying myself.

Leonard

Bolstered by Mannie's openness, Leonard, with some embarrassment, proceeded to tell his story.

Sometimes, when Rene and I are in bed for the night, she attempts to initiate sex. I find myself repelling her advances. I wonder what's wrong with me? Am I turned off by her uncharacteristic overt aggressiveness, or am I afraid that I will not be able to satisfy her? Truthfully, she's no longer the same women I married. What I've been doing to avoid the encounter is turning my back on her even though I realize it's such a cruel thing to do. I'm really ashamed of my behavior.

Even though most of the members of the group expressed sympathy and understanding, others were uncharacteristically silent during this discussion on sexuality. For many, openly sharing this intimate aspect of a relationship is definitely out of their comfort zone. The sobering restraint was natural and respected.

The frankness and the willingness of these courageous caregivers to reveal their emotions will hopefully strike a chord for some of you. Possibly it will initiate an opening for you to consider and understand your feelings about this profound deprivation in your own life.

Coping with the loss of sexuality and companionship in your relationship is difficult. An important natural part of your relationship has changed. You find yourself living in limbo with someone who looks the same but is now experienced differently. Your needs for attention and affection have not changed. But your spouse, who reacts in a regressed and childlike way, has difficulty even dressing or undressing and going to the bathroom, can no longer fill that emotional chasm.

We've observed that there are many different reactions to the loss of sexual intimacy. For some of you, as difficult as it is to deal with your personal loss, you continue to tend to your loved one's need for attention and nurturing with dedication and love. For others, fulfilling this basic human need—the desire and longing to physically and emotionally indulge in a sanctioned sexual activity with your spouse—leads to shame and guilt. You question who you are and what you're made of and wonder where you fit in. Others of you contemplate a socially unsanctioned affiliation with someone else so that the seemingly interminable loneliness and longing are eased.

EXTRAMARITAL COMPANIONSHIP

Because the progressive loss of the relationship and the accompanying feelings of loneliness become more intense as the illness continues, we will revisit this discussion on companionship as it evolves in Part 3.

What follows are some excerpts from caregivers that center on their longing for and experiences with a companion.

Nate

> I've met another woman whom I've begun to date occasionally. I know some of you may be horrified and judge my actions, but I'm so damned lonely. I love Flora very much, and I'll always take good care of her. I feel guilty. But I was getting so lonely that I was beginning to be of no practical use to Flora. I felt as if I was sinking into a deep melancholy. One evening at my pal Pete's house, I met a friend of his and we hit it off immediately. She has been widowed for almost two years. We enjoy each other's company so much. We talk as if there's no tomorrow, and I realize how long it's been since Flora and I have had any kind of meaningful conversation. Although we haven't been sexual yet, I feel closer to her every day. I don't know why I'm telling you all of this. I guess I need to vent or maybe even to receive some encouragement or feedback from you. Apart from caring for my wife, this has become one of the most complex and burdensome struggles with which I've been faced.

Jenny

Jenny's experience with an extramarital friendship presented even more complexity.

> Daily, Jenny went to the nursing home to visit her husband, Chuck, who was near the end stages of Alzheimer's. Over time, her brief conversations with a gentleman named Ned,

whose wife had been placed in the same facility just three months before, developed into a friendship. They began going out to dinner or to a movie, after they had fed their spouses. By the time Jenny's husband died, her relationship with Ned was quite serious. They became intimate and were essentially living together, either at his house or hers. During this same time, Ned was feeling a spiritual void and he returned to his church. After several months he spoke with his pastor about his relationship with Jenny. Ned told him about his confused feelings; the grief he felt for his wife's condition and the happiness he was finding with Jenny. The minister was intractable and unforgiving of Ned's behavior. Ned, after all, was living in sin and committing an immoral act in his minister's mind.

From one six-month visit that I'd made to Jenny's to the next, she had gone from ebullience and optimism to becoming forlorn and dispirited. I asked her what had changed. She told me of Ned's conversation with the pastor. Overwhelmed by guilt, Ned told her he wanted a platonic relationship with her until his wife died. Jenny made every effort to accommodate this redirection of the relationship but found it was impossible. Jenny found it both illogical and false to be forced to withhold her emotions and affection. At times she felt disingenuous. There was no satisfactory middle ground, and although both were miserable, they had decided to no longer see each other.

CHAPTER 12

Harvesting Your Communal Garden: Preventing Burnout

Previously we've mentioned the importance of maintaining your own identity and not becoming consumed by the role of caregiver. Time-outs are not selfish. If the metaphor of a well is applied to the caregiver, what comes to mind is that the well, by continually quenching the thirst of others, can run dry. Unless the heavy dark clouds burst with rain and the water seeps deep into the earth, replenishing the well, it has nothing left to give. The difference is that you, the caregiver, can influence and have control over your own emptiness. You don't have to wait passively for the heavens to open up. You do need to recognize when your "well" is running dry and decide on how to replenish yourself. Just as the rain eventually fills the empty well, so, too, does a hiatus from caregiving restore the depleted self and nurture the soul.

TAKING TIME OUT FOR YOURSELF

We can't stress enough the importance of your own self-awareness. Avoiding burnout means taking time to do whatever it is that not only provides respite but also nourishes you. Sound impossible? Some caregivers have learned to sustain themselves by taking one step at time, perhaps asking a family member, friend, or neighbor to watch their loved one for a few hours while they get out of the house to shop, play a round of golf, or meet with a friend. Others have brought someone in from a home health-care service on a regular basis for one or more days a week. Without outside help, some caregivers have made the choice to lock themselves in their bedroom or other sanctuary, where they can read, write, relax, and even catch up on some sleep. Although hesitant at first, some caregivers are able to emancipate themselves from their confining, around-the-clock duties. It is then that they report feeling less encumbered and more restored and have the necessary energy to cope again. Taking time out heals you momentarily. So when you begin to feel tired and crabby again, be aware, for it is the red flag waving again. The message: "It's time to take care of yourself."

In addition, there have been caregivers who have thought deeply about who they are and what they need to do to feel fulfilled in their lives at this time. Often, just knowing and trusting that your loved one is being adequately cared for allows you to permit yourself to take up activities that were once meaningful that you had put aside while enmeshed in the myriad tasks of caregiving. What activity would you like to reintroduce into your life that gives you pleasure and a sense of identity, a self, an "I am" beyond your caregiving role? Are there new interests or hobbies in which you would like to be involved? As difficult as it seems, it is possible and so important to find a few hours a week to play once again. Too often, we hear the following statements:

"Ooh, I cannot take being stuck at home and caring for Joe one more day!"

"I don't like the way I'm feeling lately. I'm short-tempered, impatient, and close to tears much of the time. I wish I knew what is happening to me."

"Rene is becoming a handful: she shadows me constantly and undoes whatever I've done. It's driving me nuts."

"Hazel and I almost came to blows. She doesn't understand how to do anything for herself anymore. I've been yelling at her, and last week I became so angry I almost hit her. When she started to cry, I felt so remorseful. I'm so ashamed of the way I acted, but I'm just all knots inside."

These commonly heard statements are red flags. They are clearly telling you to pay attention to such thoughts and complaints. Their message is directing you to modify and diversify how you are managing yourself in your daily activities. When you feel increasingly irritable, agitated, impatient, anxious, tearful, and out of control, these are often overt and perilous signs of burnout. Some behaviors that might alert you to burnout are yelling, rough handling of your loved one, neglect of your needs and your patient's, change in your sleep patterns and appetite, thoughts of suicide, and increased use of medications or alcohol. Any of these signs is a clue that you are not taking care of yourself, and that your needs are not being met. Consequences on your health and your patient's well-being could be severe. Caregiving is a high-stress occupation. Health problems, such as stomach ailments, heart problems, high blood pressure, depression, and bodily aches and pains, become exacerbated and immunity is compromised when you are exposed to continually stressful situations.

As caregivers you need to be cognizant that changes in your feelings, behaviors, and physical health are very significant. Give yourself permission to take time to recompose. Again, we urge you to reach out to family, friends, a caregivers' group, or a therapist for support in finding a solution. You must realize that something has to change and that there are many positive options and choices you can make. Some solutions might involve day care, in-home care, or other creative ways of achieving peace and privacy if you're confined to staying home.

DAY CARE

Jan

When I first met Jan she seemed very confident and reasonable, and I thought there might not be a time when stress would get the better of her. At this visit, however, she looked beat. She explained that Bob was still competent in many ways but was constantly shadowing her during the day and had been getting up nightly and wandering around the house. Jan tried to sleep through his wandering but woke one morning to find the refrigerator door wide open, and another morning the front door was ajar. After that, when he was up, she was up. She had unwittingly gotten into a pattern of not only being mentally spent during the day, but also having disrupted sleep every night.

On my most recent visit, it was immediately apparent to me that Jan looked noticeably different—the dark circles under her eyes had disappeared and she looked relaxed.

> I don't know how I lost sight of my own well-being, but I had, and it took a visit from my sister to finally realize what was happening. She not only let me know that I looked a wreck, but also insisted that I promise her that I would do something about it. I now have Bob in day care three days a week, but it wasn't easy even after I decided I really had to do it. Bob and I talked about day care, but he was adamantly opposed, saying he didn't want to go and was fine at home. I finally coaxed him into going, just for a visit, and he reluctantly agreed. When we got there I felt the idea was doomed. Bob saw all the other patients; many much farther along than he was in the illness, and he looked so pained I just wanted to turn around and go home, relinquishing the whole idea of day care. The director, who knew we were coming, saw us

> standing there in obvious distress and approached us, saying, "Bob, these people could really use your help. Jan told me how good you are with crafts and using tools." Well, Bob just lit up. Somewhere in him he seemed to still understand how important it was to feel needed, helpful, or to be able to contribute. In his calm way, he said that he'd be happy to help. Now he actually looks forward to going, seems much more content and is certainly more useful there than he has been at home. He does help those who are worse off than he is. Bob comes home very tired and sleeps through the night now. After feeling so lousy and having so much inner turmoil about placing Bob in day care, I'm really glad it's working out. I've rebounded and feel so much like my old self even after just these two weeks.

Nate

Nate's tall, slender body seemed bent and his shoulders drooped. His thick gray hair was in disarray, and behind his glasses his blue eyes had a desperate quality. In a clearly agitated mood he sat down. He couldn't wait to talk and fairly quickly blurted out his quandary in a voice overwrought with emotion.

> Last Friday I lost control. I blew it. Before I could stop myself, I shoved Flora so hard that she lost her balance and fell backward, hitting the bed, and then landed on the carpet. I immediately rushed to her, and here we both were kneeling on the floor hugging each other and crying together. I'm finding it harder and harder to cope. Lately I've had difficulty getting a good night's sleep. I finally drift off, but then I awaken early feeling very anxious and irritable before the day has even begun. I've become so short-tempered. Flora is really hard to deal with. She gets on a jag and asks

> me the same questions over and over again. In the late afternoon she's restless and paces and demands that we "go home." I have to take her to the bathroom constantly and am afraid not to. It's wearing me out. I'm at the end of my tether. I simply can't do this anymore.

The group members were as supportive as ever. Some, who had been in a similar situation, were especially empathetic and offered him words of comfort and advice.

> Yvette piped up, "Have you thoughtof day care at the Jewish Community Center? Their program is structured and safe. For my Richard it's a lot more interesting than the same old daily routine we have at home. You know, I was getting worn out trying to keep him amused and stimulated. His concentration span is so short; I was on the go constantly. Day care is marvelous."
>
> Bill offered a different suggestion: "How about getting someone in for a few hours a day? Someone who could be a companion for Flora. That would give you time to go out and do something for yourself. I have a lady who comes for four hours four times a week. She talks with Hazel and takes her for walks. She also picks up around the house and sometimes prepares dinner for us. I know I'm not ready to place my Hazel, and this is a good alternative. You know, we really should try to get in a round of golf sometime."
>
> As some group members tossed out similar ideas, Nate listened, taking down names of helpers he could call and also the names of various day-care centers. A calm came over his face as he realized that instead of judgment about his behavior there was encouragement, compassion, and suggested solutions. Nate realized that he did have some choices and that he could take charge of what was becoming a desperate situation for him.

A few weeks later, Nate, noticeably less troubled and more composed, told the members that he had decided to try day care.

> As one of you suggested, I didn't tell my wife ahead of time that we were going to day care. I was feeling very anxious and guilty—like I was dumping her in a strange place to get rid of her. However, after we arrived, I could tell that Flora felt important and very welcome. It's been two weeks now, and Flora seems happy there. I've had two days alone each week and have been able to catch up on sleep and some chores. I'm also contemplating having meals delivered a few times a week. Thanks to you all, I'm feeling so much better and I'm about ready to take you up on that round of golf, Bill.

Placement in day care is not always an immediate success and sorting out one's feelings around the issue not an easy task. The following stories will give you more perspective on the issues surrounding placement.

Jane

Jane was soft-spoken, somewhat unsure of herself, and definitely did not like to rock the boat. In contrast, her husband, Mac, an ex-FBI agent, was domineering, controlling, and aggressive. These traits were exacerbated by his dementia. Since Mac had stated that he did not belong in a place with old people and loonies, Jane equated placing him in day care with being a bad wife and going against her husband's wishes. Feeling overwhelmed and burned out, she finally made the decision to try it. However, three weeks later, she sat at the end of the table, somewhat chagrined, and spoke to the group.

> I decided to take Mac out of day care. Every time I get us ready to go in the morning, Mac puts up a horrible fuss and balks at

> having to go. It's becoming more difficult to get him into and out of the car. Although the staff as well as other caregivers at day care told me that Mac joined in all the activities and seemed to be having a good time, I can no longer put up with what it takes to get him there. He's been home this week and, poor man, he's trying so hard to be good, but he is still shadowing me, repeating questions, and, quite frankly, driving me nuts. I can't concentrate and I'm not getting anything done.

Yvette, picking up on Jane's feelings of failure, offered the following:

> I found it hard to get Richard to day care, too. Wow, the rows we would have in the car. He would tell me that he was not going to that place, and I would firmly tell him that he had to, and that I needed time to take care of other business. I felt so frustrated that I also considered taking him out of day care. When one of the staff told me that every day after lunch, Rich would stand at the front door and ask them when I was coming to get him, I realized that he must be feeling insecure and worried that I may abandon him. Of course he couldn't voice these fears to me. Since Rich can still tell the time, I decided to have him take his alarm clock to day care and told him that I would be there at three o'clock. That seemed to do the trick. When he finally got to the point where he could no longer tell the time, he had settled into the routine of day care.

Carolyn, energetic and self-sufficient, was a great role model. She was determined to get through her caregiving days with an upbeat attitude. She and her husband, John, had had a "good innings" (a long and happy marriage) as she said in her English accent. When John showed signs of incontinence, Carolyn felt forced to place him in day care. She spent many months researching facilities and examining her feelings before she took the huge step. The process was filled with anguish and anxiety. So often this is a profoundly difficult step to take and you grieve yet another loss. However, like Carolyn, you show great courage as you marshal your inner resources to take care of the next step. She explained the following.

> I finally took John to the day-care center yesterday. One mistake I made is that I didn't heed your wise words. Those of you experienced with getting your spouses to day care had suggested that I not let him know where he was going until the last minute. Well, I told him after supper and the poor man tossed and turned all night long. He told me he hadn't slept well. I called the day-care center in the morning to warn them about his mood. I think I was half hoping that they would suggest I bring him another day, but they told me to bring him anyway, assuring me that they would attend to him and help him feel at home. What really helped was that my pal, Sheila, picked us both up on her way to take her Ken to day care. We hoped that commuting together would make the transition smoother for both John and myself. Although he was anxious and initially said that he didn't want to go, he noticed that Ken was in the backseat and willingly joined him. As Ken began to tell him all about the place, Sheila saw the tears running down my cheeks and gave my hand a squeeze. I still felt teary when I arrived back home. The house seemed so empty and quiet. I allowed myself to indulge in a brief pity party and just let it all out. When I finally composed myself, I had an uninterrupted cup of coffee and read the paper. Then I enjoyed a tranquil, long, leisurely bath. I don't remember when I've last done that. I began to acknowledge that John was in good hands. I was so happy to see him that evening. He was really tired out from all the activities, but I had renewed energy and felt so loving toward him. I think we've turned a significant corner here, but the entire experience leading up to and through that first day was much more difficult than I thought it would be.

Leonard had placed his wife Rene in a day-care center one-and-a-half years ago.

When I think back to the time when I decided to place Rene, I realize that what made the decision so monumental for me was that I wasn't ready to let go of her. It was my problem. I've had such a hard time acknowledging that Rene needed more than I could give her. All of the excuses that I came up with to keep her at home! She's not ready for day care. She's not as sick as the others are. She'll hate it there and hate me, too. She'll think I'm deserting her.

This was not about Rene. It was all about me and my fears and reluctance to admit that I could no longer handle her on my own. And yet, I was beginning to feel resentful. I had no time to myself. I was sleeping poorly and sometimes forgetting to give Rene her medication. What really helped me take some action and think more clearly was listening to those of you who also didn't make this decision lightly. You helped me separate out whether it was Rene who was not ready or me. Thank you, my friends. I think Rene and I are doing okay.

IN-HOME CARE

Acknowledging once again that each and every one of you has different feelings, belief systems, preferences, and life circumstances, we know that day care may not seem like a good fit for you. What we want to encourage is the idea that you have a choice. Once you are cognizant of this and open to options, you will again feel empowered. If day care is not your preference but you need respite, there are other possibilities. Home care is one very realistic alternative.

Elsie

Even though Elsie was a younger caregiver, her fibromyalgia prevented her from having the energy to consistently care for her husband and household. Although she struggled with her mixed emotions—feeling somewhat the failure, having concerns about loss of privacy, and worrying about outside help being trustworthy and competent—she felt forced to hire someone.

> When Lucia arrived at the door, I was a little surprised. She looked like a little teenager, and I was sure I'd made a big mistake. I gave Lucia the lay of the land and told her that Fred was cooperative and capable of performing basic tasks with assistance. She would need to help him with bathing, shaving, dressing, and using the bathroom. I also told Lucia that Fred never seemed to have enough to do, and I was wearing myself out trying to keep him active. Lucia listened and then went right to Fred. She really knew how to engage him and had boundless energy and patience. Besides overseeing all of his activities of daily living, Lucia would take him for walks and garden with him, and when Fred was relaxing in front of the television, she would do some of the more strenuous household chores for me. I could rest when I needed to or run errands, which had become so difficult to do with Fred. As Fred got worse, Lucia's hours got longer and longer. In fact, she began to spend the night and care for him when he wandered or was restless. I know things don't always work out so beautifully for everyone, but Lucia has really been like a heavenly gift for us.

Bill

Bill was a remarkable caregiver and a devoted husband. Although he struggled with caregiving issues, he always had a smile and a joke to share with the group. He also seemed more adaptable to the changing roles and would tell the group it was because his mother made him learn to cook and iron and do those "girlie" chores when he was still a young sprout living at home. When Hazel fell and broke her hip, Bill was forced to hire an in-home health provider.

I'd been caring for Hazel fairly well up till a month ago, but since she broke her hip and is laid up, I don't get anything done. Hazel's constantly calling for me to help her to get up and out of bed, and needing to be turned. I have to be vigilant all the time. I'm afraid if I don't go to her when she calls, she might try to get up on her own and we'd have a real disaster. I came to a decision that I really needed help. We interviewed several people, and my wife seemed to be taken with a young woman by the name of Cynthia. She talked with Hazel and asked her some questions. Although Hazel would mostly reply in gibberish, Cynthia would respond appropriately. That sold me. Cynthia has come now for four days, and it's made such a difference to us. I wonder why I didn't get help sooner. My wife seems to perk up when Cynthia's there, and I'm feeling so much better. Cynthia's very gentle with Hazel, and gets her up and out of the house in her wheelchair every day. Oh yes, what a relief it is. Now I can work on my computer and get to the other business around the house. You know—those girlie chores and all. Practically speaking, I've always been very conservative with my finances. My kids have another word for it. They just call me cheap. This may have been another reason that really got in the way of my making this decision. Home care is not free by any means. But depending on how this crazy illness goes, I think I can handle it financially. If not, as much as I would hate to do it, my kids have offered to pitch in. Right now it's a lot cheaper than paying for my stay in the loony bin.

GOING IT ALONE

For philosophical or financial reasons, many caregivers decide to continue caring for their spouse without help from the outside. Even though there is a sense of autonomy and mastery in doing this, the danger is in not taking time for yourself. What follows are some creative ways that homebound caregivers found prevented them from being engulfed by the influences of burnout.

Joy

> I've always had a passion for reading. As caregiving became more tedious and emotionally draining, reading was my escape. However in Ned's mid-stages of Alzheimer's, finding the time and a quiet space became impossible for me until I remembered back to when our children were toddlers. I would put myself in the playpen and read while allowing them the rest of the house. It seemed imperative that I reclaim that metaphoric playpen. I asked myself, "What is the worst thing that could happen if I hide for two hours?" I thought of all of the dangers I would need to eliminate. I safety latched all of the outside doors, put out some finger food, and set the VCR to play videos of old Westerns and nature shows for Ned. Then I went to the bedroom and closed the door behind me, promising myself that I would stay there for two hours. Ned was fine with this plan. However, it took me several days to be able to relax and not feel compelled to check up on Ned every fifteen minutes. Now I do enjoy my quiet time in my "playpen" and have read some wonderful books.

Herb

Herb decided he would claim that metaphoric "space" by writing his wife's biography.

> I was very fortunate that Jean was never aggressive or combative throughout her battle with Alzheimer's. For a long period

in the course of her illness, Jean would nap after lunch and I could sit at my old Royal typewriter and retrace her life from stories she had told me and from my own recollections. I knew the finality of her illness and the transitions that had already muted her personality. I wanted our children to know and never forget their mother, as she once was—the young farm girl, the army nurse, the saxophone player, and the righteous feminist. I wanted them to remember her beauty, her "joie de vivre," her tenderness and strength. I wanted to include photographs, and when I got out the boxes of pictures and albums to select a few, I found that Jean would spend hours going through them. This was an unexpected and wonderful outcome. Writing the book was not only a gift to our children, but the process gave me tremendous peace and joy.

Olga

For years, especially when money was tight after the war, I supplemented our family income as a seamstress. It wasn't only a profession I could base at home, which was important when our kids were young, but I enjoyed my role in sharing the excitement and planning of my clients' special occasions. I can remember every wedding dress I made down to the last bead. With this profession I also had the flexibility of arranging my schedule to fit in with my family's needs. Now that I must stay home with Gus, my sewing brings the outside in once again. I'm even making wedding gowns for some of my old clients' daughters. I can work at my own pace doing something that always gave me pleasure and a sense of fulfillment. With the money I earn, I'm saving up to go on a splurge with my daughters to Hawaii—someday.

CHAPTER 13

I Think I Can, I Think I Can, I Know I Can: Resiliency

Throughout the duration of your years as caregivers, most of you have told us how surprised you were at yourselves for being able to get through it all, weathering the crises, caprice, and unpredictability. You are really quite a sturdy lot. The role of caregiver is complex and challenging, but you've proved it's not inscrutable. Caregiving is a jolt, a lightening bolt that strikes and forces you to change your habitual and customary role, lifestyle, and relationship not only with your spouse but with yourself as well. As you will observe, so many like you have mastered the challenge. Resiliency is the key to victory over Alzheimer's disease.

In one of our group discussions, we focused on abilities and strengths the members had developed or rediscovered in themselves through their caregiving experiences.

The question was asked, "As you look back over the course of your caregiving encounters and ordeals so far, how have you changed, what have you learned, and how have you grown in this role?"

When Jane first joined the group, over two years ago, she always appeared tense, with her lips drawn and her jaw set. In answering the question, Jane, her face relaxed and composed, smiled from ear to ear as she spoke.

> It's a big shift from having to prove you're right at any cost, to communicating with an Alzheimer's patient where being right becomes superfluous, useless. When I think back to the beginning of Mac's illness, and how I reacted to everything, I feel so much better about myself today. Instead of arguing, I agree with everything that he says, whether he's right or wrong. I used to be so bull-headed about how right I was, and we would carry on like kids. I'd yell to him and he'd yell back, it soon became a competition—which one of us could yell the loudest. Then we would both stomp off feeling rotten, and nothing was resolved. I've finally learned to keep my big mouth shut and not argue. I say to myself repeatedly "don't argue, don't argue." With time and practice it's getting easier. As I said, I'll either go along with what Mac says, or I may tell him that I will think about it or distract him or even help him. Usually that satisfies him, and before long he has forgotten what he was becoming so riled up about. I've learned that I don't have to be right all the time, and in doing so have claimed an even greater victory.

Jane's insight stimulated eager responses from the group members, who all wanted a turn to share the progress they felt they had made from their initiation into caregiving to this point.

Len contributed the following.

> I don't get as worked up and angry as I used to by Rene's wild behavior. Instead of reacting, I've become more loving and patient with her. Practicing patience has been particularly difficult. And believe me it has taken practice. Counting to ten and sometimes to twenty. I found that as I became more patient I was also less exasperated. As a result I can feel more

compassion for her. I don't judge her or critically point out her mistakes. After all, she's being cheated out of life much more than I am. She would never do the things she does if her brain was functioning normally. I have to separate her from the unnerving influence of this disease.

Carolyn joined right in.

I hear you, Len, and agree with the importance of being patient. Along with that I've learned acceptance, which seemed necessary before I felt I could take control and cope. I'm not sure I could have done it though without the support of the group and my strong faith in God. I realize that I can't do any more than I'm doing. I can't change the disease, but I can change the way I think and how I choose to cope. I believe the good Lord won't give me anything I can't handle.

Angela added:

I think the word that strikes me is "change." The circumstances of Joe's illness have forced me into it, but I'm all the better for it. The illness has changed him and transformed me. I've moved from resentment to compassion and from bitterness and anger to acceptance.

Angela's face showed the strain of the deep emotion she felt, and with a break in her voice she continued.

Coming to terms with Joe's decline has not been easy.

Mannie had made it his purpose to lighten us up when the atmosphere in the room became charged and heavy. With a dimpled smile, and in his deep voice, he jumped in.

> I've made it through this illness without my knickers in a twist because of my belief in getting through life with a sense of humor. Alzheimer's is the pits, and for a time there I really started getting down. It took me a while and a conscious effort to regain my sense of humor, accommodate to this illness that was obviously here to stay, and learn to lighten up. I feel so bad for Rachel, but sometimes she does the darndest things. The other day she came to breakfast with red eye shadow and baby blue lips. Sometimes you just have to laugh.

When Elizabeth first visited the group, her voice was shaky and barely audible. She was having a rough time coping with her husband's dementia and, as with many caregivers, had become immersed and preoccupied in her caregiving role—so much so that she had isolated herself from friends and family. She felt lonely, forsaken, and depressed. It was her doctor who recommended that she attend a support group. After participating for many months, she not only began to find her voice and develop friendships, but she also became self-assured and felt truly understood. Elizabeth spoke in a soft but clear voice.

> I felt lost and isolated before I came to this group. Thanks to Mannie's humor and all of you and your unwavering encouragement, I have made deeper connections with friends, getting beyond my shyness and resistance and seeking them out. On your advice I've asked my children for help, which they were more than willing to give. I'm taking better care of myself and appreciating all that I can about Harvey and our time together during this part of our lives. I have learned that there's no reason to suffer alone, but that it was ultimately up to me to decide to change that.

Hooray to all of you!

COMING TO TERMS WITH THE CHALLENGES OF ALZHEIMER'S

Almost every caregiver has arrived, over time, at the place where they mindfully begin to acknowledge and accept the ambiguous and provocative nature of the disorder. You will, too. You'll become less perturbed and more proficient as you care for your loved one. The more you learn about strategies that you can employ, the more creative and flexible you become in dealing with various behaviors, the easier the tasks will be. You can improve your skills by reading books and educational articles about Alzheimer's behavioral problems, and by talking with a professional or with other caregivers.

Once you are able to separate the brain disease from the person who is your loved one, you will be more able to come to terms with Alzheimer's disease. You will be less likely to personalize your loved one's actions. In fact, although your moods initially will tend to rise and fall with the variability of the course of Alzheimer's disease, the lows will not seem to be as arching nor will they last as long. Part and parcel in assessing your own competency and understanding is to begin to know and acknowledge your limits and to be compassionate with yourself. A cautionary note: Be aware of mounting physical and emotional stress and take care of yourself on a daily basis so that you are able to retain your strength to proceed on this journey.

PART THREE

THE LATE MIDDLE STAGE

CHAPTER 14
The Long Goodbye

Mamie

Mamie lifted Bud's legs into the car, fastened his seatbelt, and closed the door. She then let herself in the driver's side. Bud looked at her inquisitively and said, "Where's Mamie?" Taken aback, she responded, "Bud, I'm Mamie!" He said, "No, you're not. My Mamie is much younger and prettier than you are." Mamie glanced at her image in the rearview mirror, sighed at the reflection of a woman of seventy-eight, and then became very sad. It was not the first time that Bud, in referencing the past as present, no longer recognized her as his wife, his companion of fifty years, his Mamie. This incident was a turning point for her. To Mamie, Bud was still her husband. To Bud, she could be anyone.

For the rest of the day Mamie dwelt on that interchange. She continued to ruminate as she buttoned and zipped

> Bud's pants after he used the bathroom, and then as she led him into the den and turned on the TV. Mamie was deep in thought as she cut up Bud's dinner and sat patiently with him until he finished eating, and later as she maneuvered him into bed and tucked him in for the night. She clearly realized that there was no longer the familiar, "Thanks, Mamie," or "Best meatloaf this side of the Mississippi, Lovie," or "Goodnight, Bride." Mamie sat in the darkness and cried for a long time. The realization that she was no longer a part of Bud's world became crystal clear. Physically tired and emotionally spent, she went to bed. On arising, Mamie would once again find a way to adapt to the significant change in Bud's cognition caused by Alzheimer's disease.

Up until now, you have been challenged with many adjustments and out of necessity have been forced to habituate to the disease. Entering the "late-middle" stage of Alzheimer's disease, with full awareness that there is no going back or getting better, and as tedium sets in and emotional exhaustion threatens, you will discover that you can muster extraordinary strength, courage, and stamina in order to persevere and persist.

LATE-MIDDLE-STAGE BEHAVIORS

The late-middle stage of Alzheimer's disease usually begins five or more years from onset and can go on for a long time. At this stage, your patient will no longer have the ability to think rationally or consequentially, demonstrate willpower in order to problem solve, be involved in decision making, or carry out a purposeful course of action. He or she will have only sketchy knowledge of past and present events and will possibly be unable to recognize friends and relatives, even those most familiar, and his or her own image in the mirror. Communicating with language is limited as the ability to retrieve words and speak in cogent sentences is compromised. Emotional communication is minimal.

Your spouse will need help in varying degrees with all of his or her activities of daily living: bathing and general hygiene; dressing systematically and appropriately for time, place, and weather; eating nutritiously with adequate solid and liquid intake, often needing reminders to chew and swallow.

Your patient may seem less coordinated, therefore unable to use utensils adeptly, and may display a shuffling gait when walking, therefore becoming more prone to stumbling. Bowel and bladder control may also be compromised, minimally by needing reminders or help with direction to the bathroom and with zippers, or more severely by incontinence and lack of bowel control. He or she may sleep more and have confusion as to day and night. Wandering throughout the house or "shadowing" you may become a daily pattern.

These changes, sometimes dramatic, often sneak up on you before you have realized that your spouse has deteriorated to a new stage, a different level of the disease, therefore adding significantly to the burden of caregiving. Physically caring for your patient becomes much more difficult. You may need to do more lifting, bending, and maneuvering. Moreover, it may be necessary for you to attend to your patient more often; for example, reminding him or leading him to the bathroom every two hours or so. As you assertively and effectively take over many activities that were previously in your spouse's domain, in addition to all of the household tasks and financial affairs, please be aware that your physical and emotional health are more at risk. Emotionally, you may experience feelings of anger, frustration, and resentment, which can be manifested by crying spells or other uncharacteristic behavior. Commonly, you begin to show some signs of burnout. Therefore you must be alert to the signs and symptoms that your body is giving you.

LOSS OF RECOGNITION BY SPOUSE

As we shared in Mamie's story at the beginning of this chapter, one of the most poignant outcomes in this stage of Alzheimer's is the inability of your spouse to recognize you. In your awareness of this painful reality, you acutely mourn the loss of the relationship at a deeper level. Feelings of grief intensify. Up until this time, you have been intellectually aware that this loss of recognition is an inevitable part of the illness and has been looming in the distance. Let's hope you have begun to prepare yourself for this eventuality. Many caregivers, in anticipation of this stage, begin to make statements that begin with, "when he no longer recognizes me . . . " Often followed by ". . . I will have in-home health care," or ". . . I will place her."

In a sense, you may also feel that you are in no-man's land, neither fish nor fowl. Looking back at fifteen, thirty, fifty or more years of marriage, you appreciate the relationship that was, the partnership that grew, through ups and downs, and developed in both depth and meaning. The place in which you now find yourself is somewhat paradoxical. You're married, but this union is contradictory to the defined or experienced paradigm that in essence constitutes a marriage. The familiarity and reliability of the relationship that was, and the limbo in which you now find yourselves, is something to be reckoned with. The answers are deeply rooted in man's need for a sense of belonging that identifies "who" we are and "how" we can contribute in a way that gives meaning to our lives in both substance and essence.

The missing "we," the union, the "us" who walked arm and arm together is a lamentable loss. You need time and support in order to overcome and make peace with your sorrow. To get beyond the mourning and redefine who you are and where you belong is an achievable task. In the evolution of grieving this enormous loss of both the relationship as well as your sense of self, you will find great solace and comfort in the memories of a partnership that flowered over time into a closeness and mutuality of inestimable value.

In our group setting and in-home interviews, we have many stories of experiences during this stage which caregivers refer to as "the long good-bye" and in which they begin to refer to themselves as "married widows and widowers." In sharing these stories, we hope you will be exposed to and inspired by creative ways other caregivers have found to bring meaning to their lives at this time.

Like the Chinese definition for the word "crisis"—blending challenge with opportunity—you can and will find new direction, and will continue to have a life that is meaningful. In the coming chapters, we will address solutions to some of the challenges you face in your caregiving that no longer surprise you but can take a toll, because of their unrelenting tenacity and their siege on your emotions. Through your stories we want to show you the possibilities of surviving, growing, and maintaining a healthy "self" in this continuum we call life.

CHAPTER 15

I'm Beat and I'm Scared: Caregiving Intensifies—Resource Options

A predominant issue that surfaces as tasks become more difficult and time consuming and you grow more weary, is that of letting go of the daily care of your spouse and giving up a desire for perfection and control. The belief that many cling to is that it is only you who can optimally do the job of caring for your loved one in the right way. Although a worthy concept, an unwavering commitment to this ideal can be self-sabotaging. In a desire to maintain complete control, you may become so emotionally and physically spent that you lose the sense of objectivity and clarity necessary for making the best and healthiest decisions for you and your spouse. In order to keep body and soul together, you must let go of unrealistic desire and self-flagellation. The stories told in this chapter are meaningful examples of how caregivers find the willingness to let go, use good judgment, trust their inner resources, and reach out for the love and support of friends and family.

It's a common pitfall for you as a caregiver: You become so focused on your loved one and deeply immersed in your caregiving routines, that you put your own life on hold, don't take time to reduce your stress, and compromise your own health. In the constant struggle to maintain balance in your life, you need to learn to say "I can't do this anymore, I need help."

FAMILY INVOLVEMENT

You have many options from which to choose, including help from family and friends, place of worship, and community resources, such as in-home help, day care, support groups, and government agencies. In most cities, the Alzheimer's Association is a good place to start. The association knows of the availability of various resources in each community and is often the provider of some of those services.

For each of you, the measure and kind of help will be different based on your own physical and mental health as well as your ability to satisfy the varied needs of your patient. We stress again and again in this book that Alzheimer's disease is a family problem. Keeping the family involved and responsible as caregiving becomes more difficult is paramount in importance. Research has demonstrated that caregivers who have an involved, supportive network of family and friends tend to cope much better than those who are more isolated. Children particularly need to know what's really going on so that they can participate. Some of you may actually decide to move closer to your children. Children in the same city need to reassess their own schedules in order to accommodate the needs of both parents. However, understanding that today extended families are often hundreds of miles away, regular and frequent communication providing emotional support and participation in making major decisions is vital. The tables have turned, and it is an opportunity for the children to give back.

Jane

Jane's situation provides a good example regarding children's involvement.

Jane and Mac had been married well over fifty years and had six adult children. One lived in the same town, and although the others were out of state, they were very willing to visit in order to give Jane some respite and to check on their dad and the situation at home. Jane attended the support group fairly erratically. It was difficult for her to openly share the frustrations and the pain she experienced in watching her husband as his abilities declined. She was a very private woman, and although she would give a brief description of her experiences and express her regret that she was so impatient, she would go no further, explaining to us that she wanted to respect her husband's privacy and to preserve his dignity. However, she did learn a lot by listening to what the others in the group had to say. Sometimes her daughter, Mimi, would attend the group with her. Jane had told me previously that she confided in Mimi and was open to the three of us being candid with each other in learning how to take care of Mac in the best possible way.

One day, Mimi called me aside because she was concerned that her mother was becoming increasingly frustrated and was acting in a passive-aggressive manner toward her father. She explained that Jane would needle him endlessly, and then she would become both angry with herself and overcome with guilt. We decided that if Jane were agreeable, which she was, perhaps individual therapy would allow her to talk about the impact her husband's regressive behaviors had on her. In the privacy and safety of the office, Jane was able to open up that festering wound of unacknowledged feelings and also look, for the first time, at the fact that she needed additional help in caring for Mac. We set an appointment for us to meet with Mimi in order to make some decisions. In the meeting, Jane stated that she specifically wanted a man to come into the house and take care of her husband two to three times a week. She wanted him to take Mac out for a drive or a long walk and generally keep him active. During the office visit, with the intent of allowing Jane and Mimi to take control of the situation, we concluded that they ought to investigate what the community could offer.

After calling several resources—agencies that provided in-home care, as well as the Alzheimer's Association—both Jane and Mimi interviewed several prospective male caregivers until they found one who they believed was most appropriate, in terms of his personality, to care for Mac. Jane was both relieved and grateful that she did not have to make this decision alone. Mimi's intervention and support made all the difference to Jane, and in coming to a reasonable solution. Mimi felt very good about their ability to make a decision together that improved the wellbeing of both her mother and father. Another benefit for Jane was that she felt more in control as she had deliberately planned a course of action.

Stella

In the last several months, Stella recognized that she was feeling the effects of burnout and was encouraged by her friends and family to plan a respite. Respite is one way in which you can recharge your batteries and return to the task of caregiving with renewed energy and optimism. Stella's respite worked wonders for her but also had a profound impact on her daughter.

My friend Irma wanted a companion to accompany her on an Elder Hostel's trip to the Gold Country, so, with everyone pushing me, I decided to go. Patty, my oldest, said she would

> leave the kids with her husband, Bob, and take care of her dad for the week. In our judicious planning, she arrived, we went over the schedule and her dad's needs, and I was off to the bus with Irma. The week went quickly. I had such a good time and felt so rejuvenated. However, on my return home, I immediately saw that Patty was beat, and I could tell from her puffy eyes that she had been crying. She explained that in the first place, even though I had been telling her about her dad, she had no idea how really difficult getting through the day could be, with all his little shortcomings really adding up. She said that she had had to be so patient and vigilant all the time.
>
> More poignantly, she started to cry and told me that she wasn't sure her dad even knew who she was. One evening as he stared vacantly at the television, she took his hand and held it for a long time. She looked at it and recalled that this was one of the strong and trusting hands she had known as a child. Those hands that confidently picked her up and swung her in the air as if she were weightless. She remembered her dad tentatively shaking hands with Charlie Perkins, her first date, while he looked disapprovingly at Charlie's ducktail and leather jacket, but said nothing to embarrass her. It was that same hand she was now holding that wiped her tears of joy on her graduation and led her onto the dance floor on her wedding day. I felt terrible, until she told me that this experience had been so very important for her. She was grateful not only to have had this time with her dad but also to have a better understanding of what my day-to-day life is like.

Because of this bittersweet experience, Patty was able to reconcile herself to her father's illness and reflect on how wonderful he'd been and how much he loved her. The other positive outcome was that she really understood and could empathize with what her mother's daily life was like.

Alzheimer's disease has been referred to as a "family disease." It affects everyone in the family; everyone is, in some way, changed by it. Like the disease process itself, Alzheimer's effects on family are subtle at first and then it pervades those relationships in complex ways. What often comes to the surface is how the intricacies of family relationships are played out. That is, how emotional issues as well as behaviors are dealt with. Do children and parents come together and work as a team, or do they become fragmented? Do adult children hang in there as both Stella's and Joan's daughters did, or do they turn away? Is this due to dysfunctional family relationships or because it is often too painful and scary for adult children to face the fact that their once strong and reliable parent is now weak and vulnerable? Who is it that steps into the leadership role, wanting to take control and use their power either to dominate or to make decisions that will be beneficial for all? A very relevant issue is that of grief. How do families grieve and let go of a beloved? How do they communicate their feelings about this loss? How do children support and protect the caregiving parent and vice versa?

The answers to these questions are as unique and varied as each individual in the family unit. Some families need support and guidance through this undulating maze of emotion and problem solving, while others finds the means to endure and succeed in the strength of their particular family unit. Caregiving is an enormous task to accomplish alone.

Family caregivers, and caregivers in general, who do eventually succeed are those who concede that change is inevitable in our lives. The circumstances of caregiving require that you reprioritize on a continuum and become more flexible than you probably have ever had to be. When acceding to this, many of you and your families do redefine and reshape your lives. You begin slowly, cautiously, and reluctantly to navigate in unfamiliar territory, and by the end of the journey, you may all be transformed by the experience in valuable ways that you never believed were possible. Often family ties are strengthened and relationships improve. There is more freedom to express thoughts and feelings previously unspoken. Alzheimer's becomes the catalyst for bringing the family together to work toward goals and solutions for the problems in caregiving, and to grieve together for the loss of the beloved parent and spouse.

ALTERNATIVES TO PLACEMENT

Please note that generally the word "placement" refers to the admission or entry of a patient into any care facility, and that is the term we'll use throughout the book.

In the late-middle stage of Alzheimer's, the needs of the patient may have increased to the point that having someone come in two or three days a week to relieve the caregiver is no longer adequate. Caregiving now requires meeting the basic needs around dressing, bathing, feeding, assistance with walking, and incontinence on a daily basis. You may feel exhausted and depleted.

For some of you, the idea of placement is out of the question. Whether finances, myths or realities about placement, or previous irrevocable promises made to your spouse lead to your determination to keep your spouse at home, the fact is that very few caregivers succeed single-handedly. The physical burden in itself becomes impossible to manage. On the other hand, for only a small percentage of the population is twenty-four-hour home care affordable or available. Success in keeping your loved one at home is often attained through a combination of care and intervention by family, friends, and home health aids until the final stages when hospice care becomes appropriate.

The day came when Andy had to face that he could no longer take care of Martha on his own. His back had been killing him, he wasn't sleeping properly, he was exhausted and getting depressed. It was apparent from the outset that in his mind, placement was not an option, even though it had been suggested more than once.

Andy

Mary, I'm just not going to do it. I watched Mom die in one of those places and have regretted it to this day. It's not going to happen to Martha. I promised her and myself that she would never end up in a nursing home. You could tell me a hundred times, "just go and take a look," but I'm not going to do it. My daughter has said the same thing, Mary, so no offense. She and I are going to work it out.

And work it out they did. At first Andy took complete care of Martha, and his daughter, Judy, who had gone back to college recently agreed to come in to help several evenings a week with the laundry, cleaning, and cooking. As his caregiving intensified, Andy worked hard to keep up with the constant pressures, but the stress and physical strain were evident over the course of time. His back ached and his mood darkened. He had stopped meeting with his buddies that he'd known for years at the Model Railroad Club. Judy decided to cut back on her classes and come over during the day, three times a week and on the weekends. Andy felt guilty that Judy would be prolonging her studies toward her degree, but Judy insisted that her mother's care was both of their responsibilities. Toward the end of Martha's illness, Andy asked Martha's physician to order hospice care at home, and for the first time in months, Andy could sleep, eat, and rest with his mind at ease. Keeping Martha at home came with a price; a toll taken on Andy's health and an isolation that he really didn't anticipate. But would he or his daughter have had it any other way? Never.

Gil

Andy was remarkable in accomplishing his resolution not to place Martha and in personally taking on a great deal of the burden for her care. Gil, who was a hard-driving, obstinate, and aggressive businessman, loved his wife no less than Andy loved his, but he knew his own limitations. Having the resources, he chose what he felt was the best arrangement for the care of his wife.

As Phyllis's Alzheimer's progressed, Gil, an estate planner, had come to acknowledge an enormous change in their very active social life, which they both enjoyed immensely. He missed terribly the presence of his wife at his side, with her engaging conversation and effervescent smile. He always kidded that she was really the reason they had a social life at all, and he was only invited as her escort. As Phyllis's memory deteriorated further, Gil was having problems with his own concentration, to the point that he felt it was affecting his responsibilities to his clients and their portfolios. He was constantly preoccupied with Phyllis's safety. Retiring was a possibility, but he felt completely incompetent to care for Phyllis. Instinctively, he knew that he was not cut out to be a caregiver and couldn't even imagine this role. Gil reluctantly employed a full-time nurse, who moved into the bedroom next to his wife's so that Phyllis would have the constant care that she needed. Although Gil was still deeply aggrieved by his wife's deterioration, having the nurse provided the stability that gave him freedom from constant worry. Thus, he could continue with his business and community involvement. For Gil it was the best of a bad bargain, and he was really never able to completely come to terms with this horrible illness that had robbed Phyllis of her enjoyment of her children, grandchildren, and the remaining time they had together.

WHEN PLACEMENT BECOMES NECESSARY

Over time, all of the caregivers in the group would meet their Waterloo—the end of their ability to care for their spouse—each with a variation on a few familiar themes.

Mannie, who had a heart condition, was getting up every two hours to take his wife to the bathroom so she would not wet the bed—sometimes she did anyway. He was exhausted and his health was in serious jeopardy.

Angela would find herself yelling at Joe out of her own frustration and exhaustion. She would then have terrible remorse and guilt, remonstrating herself for lacking compassion. She had tried so hard to protect and preserve Joe's dignity and respect but now was finding herself consistently berating him.

Nate was on the verge of physically abusing his wife. He'd have the urge to push her into bed instead of assisting her. He was becoming lax about making sure she was drinking enough liquid and eating her meals. The day he noticed black-and-blue marks on her arms where he had grabbed her too tightly to put her out of his way in the kitchen, he sat down at the table and cried.

As these examples indicate, the decision to place your spouse is heart wrenching and complex. In fact, it may be one of the hardest decisions you will have to make. Around this issue, you will experience many mixed emotions. You may feel anxious, depressed, ashamed, or guilty as you perceive that placing your spouse in a nursing home is abandoning him or her and giving up on your commitment to care for him or her. Many of you may believe that you are the only one able to care for and meet all the needs of your family member who is suffering from dementia.

There is often an internal conflict over letting go—giving up control of your spouse—and the irrational but real anxiety over your belief that once your spouse is placed, you will become helpless and incapable of influencing the care he or she receives. Some of you who have made a promise to your spouse that you would never "put him away" in a nursing home, may now struggle with the choice of breaking that promise in spite of the necessity and practicality of placement.

Like many caregivers, it is likely that you will feel very vulnerable, as your trust in your judgment wavers and you question whether you are making the right decision. Ideally, the decision to place your loved one should be made as a family. When you have support, your vacillation and ambivalence are replaced with more certainty and acceptance. This involvement will strengthen the family's cohesiveness and ease your burden. More often than not, it is the family that encourages making this decision before the caregiver is ready to do so. However, when the family is reticent or there is discord about the placement of their parent, often outside intervention is necessary to support that decision or to plan alternatives that protect your health and well-being.

In the case of caregivers who do not have family members they can count on or turn to, it becomes even more critical to reach out to friends or community for guidance. This is one time when members of a support group can act in the role of an extended family and offer suggestions, empathy, and, most of all, encouragement that comes from the heart of their own experiences.

Elizabeth

At Elizabeth's request, and her children's insistence, a family session was conducted in the privacy of my office. Present in the session were Elizabeth, her four adult children, and their spouses. One of her daughters lived close by, and the others lived out of state. Her children had expressed concern about their mother. The stimulus for their anxiety and apprehension was their mother's unusual behavior. Elizabeth was exhibiting signs of caregiver burnout: angry outbursts; resentment toward her husband, Harvey; indecisiveness; irritation; and fatigue. To her children's amazement, their mother, who was normally controlled and kept her emotions in check, would have uncontrollable crying spells. The children described that she would instigate fights with Harvey and then castigate him. Again, very much out of character. The result of these provocations on Harvey, was that he suffered further loss of self-esteem and his sadness increased.

> We rallied around the table to problem solve. Although all of the children were worried, they were not in agreement about the amount or kind of care their father needed. One of the children who lived out of state was still in denial that his father needed help at all. Elizabeth's closest daughter was really pushing for additional in-home help. It was important

for Elizabeth's children, as well as for Elizabeth, to understand the underlying dynamics of her increasingly harsh and uncharacteristic behavior and to recognize the importance of taking action. It was also essential to use this forum in order to decide what would be in both parents' best interest, and especially Mom, who was the sole caregiver.

Harvey had been an attorney, a very capable and dependable man whom Elizabeth loved and respected. She had often turned to him to share an experience or to ask for his opinion and views on a subject. The children recalled their memories about their father, which aligned with those of their mother. He was a father whom they admired, respected, and felt they could go to for sage advice. Discussion centered a lot on the loss of these relationships and the emotional effect it was having on Elizabeth as well as the adult children.

Being willing and able to talk about issues openly served as a valuable, cathartic experience for all present. They had not shared their fears, feelings of loss, and frustrations with one another. Paradoxically, this family meeting, although painful, had the very positive effect of firmly binding their kinship. Their tears acted as a catalyst for releasing the inner torment they were experiencing and for sharing intense and painful feelings with each other. All too often in families, members remain silent because they do not want to rock the boat, talk about the unspeakable. Or, as in this family, some members were not able to cope with their raw and grievous emotions and denied the reality of the situation they faced.

The positive release of complex and competing emotions could only be attained in a structured, safe setting where a neutral third party could take on the helpful role of therapist or mediator. Each person was directed to speak only for himself and had the opportunity to hold the floor without interruption so that the others could listen to and possibly resonate with what was being expressed. This way of interacting, in which respect for one another's views was paramount to the success of the meeting, allowed the formerly splintered group to eventually come to an agreement by which they could all abide. In this nonvolatile setting, they found the courage to cautiously project and propose possible future plans of action. They realized that this could mean full-time in-home help for their parents or placement of their father. Elizabeth, having expressed her strong desire to keep Harvey at home throughout his illness, had been heard—another all-too-heavy burden lifted from her shoulders. The practicalities of this decision were openly debated, the pros and cons measured. Elizabeth and her family agreed to keep Harvey at home for as long as possible. There was also consensus that they would research and visit suitable nursing homes in order to be prepared for the future. Ultimately, the decision to place Harvey presented itself and the family met again in order to support their mother and each other through this sad and trying transition.

THE ANGST OF PLACEMENT

There is no more difficult a decision for you than that of placing your spouse in a facility. The significance of this physical separation and relinquishing control as the primary caregiver is immense, and feelings of loss, mourning, guilt, and self-recrimination often accompany the decision.

For almost all of you, there does come a time when taking care of your spouse in your home becomes, in reality, too difficult to continue. Those of you who have utilized resources such as day care, in-home care, or respite have already taken some action involving physical separation. This may make the adjustment to permanent placement somewhat less traumatic. You've begun to let go of control of daily care for your spouse and have begun to accommodate the idea of having your loved one in a care facility. In spite of this "preparation," caregivers have said that the feelings of loss are still profound.

Because placement may be the first time that you as a couple are actually living apart physically, this loss involves a deeper bereavement than any experienced up to this time in the course of your spouse's Alzheimer's disease. Aware and heartsore that your loved one will never be returning home, you experience emotional turmoil that is at a more spiritual and soul-felt level. Where there was once a person who was there in the morning when you awakened or turned around or sat down or turned out the light, or whose shadow cast a long familiar figure on the sidewalk alongside of yours, there is now a void. You're reminded that it's time to accommodate, yet again, to a different stage of the disease. Another plateau to which you had grown accustomed has changed, and the end of one stage is now the beginning of a more profoundly different one in your journey as caregiver. You question your own identity. Who am I now that I've relinquished my role as primary caregiver? I'm married, but how is this marital relationship defined? Many caregivers refer to themselves at this point as "married widows and widowers." You're faced with the challenge of redefining the life role that you will play, one in which you will find the most meaning and satisfaction. Remember that the result of caregiving and grieving is often an initiation into a deeper, more meaningful life experience.

Angela

Friends ask me how come I'm so tired during the day, even though Joe is in day care. Well, let me tell you why. When Joe would return from day care, I'd have to pump myself up in order to find the energy and internal fortitude to get through the long night that lay ahead. I knew that I'd have to be with him every minute. Usually I'd have dinner ready and sit with Joe for at least an hour while he ate. I'd watch him as he slowly and laboriously put every bite of food on his fork. He would chew and chew and chew. I would remind him to swallow and try to make sure that he did. I'd hold his glass of water for him so that he could drink. The doctor told me to make sure that Joe was getting plenty of liquid. That, in itself, was hard. Sometimes using a straw would work best and other times he'd do well with a baby cup that had a spout. I wouldn't even try to clean the dishes afterward, as Joe insisted on helping and it just doubled the work.

Getting Joe ready for bed was the worst. He'd become very

obstinate, and I'd have to struggle to get him out of his clothes and into his pajamas. I'd try to help him brush his teeth, but sometimes he'd refuse to open his mouth. Once I'd settled him into bed for the night, he'd often be in and out of it three or four times. Because he'd forget how to get back in again, I'd have to grit my teeth as I called on every ounce of patience I had to get him settled again. It's hard to believe how much time this takes and what a physical workout it is. You really have to watch how you're lifting and bending or you'll get it in the back.

Sometimes, Joe would sleep through the night and other times he wouldn't. Of course, I was awake every time he was. Then, at the crack of dawn, we'd be up in order to have him ready for the van that picked him up and took him to day care. Dressing him was like dressing a 170-pound doll. I grew to hate socks. I would feed him breakfast and rush to get him to the curb in time for the van to pick him up. At least the driver would help me get Joe into the van. Then I'd go back to bed for a few hours and try to sleep.

In spite of reminding myself over and over that it was this dreadful disease and not Joe that was causing my anger and frustration, I got to the point with Joe where I was snapping at him, yelling, and feeling angry and resentful much of the time. That is when I knew deep in my heart that it was time to place him in a nursing facility. I didn't want to, but when I asked myself how much good am I for him these days, when I am so tired and bad tempered, I honestly couldn't say that I was being of any use to either one of us. When Joe first went to day care, I sent him one day a week and soon increased it to two, then three, and eventually he was attending day care five to six times a week. Now even this was not enough. I tried to take care of him at home as long as I could. I just couldn't do it any longer.

Even though Angela was about at her breaking point, placing Joe was still an extremely difficult decision to make. She couldn't imagine Joe no longer sleeping in bed next to her, or sitting in the lounge chair across from hers in the living room of an evening, or sharing meals together at the little table in the kitchen. She could not envision Joe simply not being there. For a long time now, Angela had resisted taking the step of placing Joe, clearly understanding how permanent this relocation would be for him. For her, it was a last resort, a giant step that she now felt forced to take.

Ogden

Ogden's decision making around placing Adele differed somewhat from Angela's. His physical health was jeopardizing his ability to take care of Adele. It isn't unusual to find that your health might be more fragile than that of your Alzheimer's spouse.

> Ogden was a grand gentlemen's gentleman who had an infectious optimism and benevolence toward everyone. He adored his wife, Adele, and as he saw her decline, he worried that he wouldn't be able to care for her once she became incapable of performing the activities of daily living. He had a prosthetic leg, which was really quite unreliable when it came to lifting or otherwise assisting his wife, and more recently he had had two transient ischemic attacks (TIAs, or ministrokes). He called on his son to give him a helping hand in finding a three-tier facility that could accommodate both himself and Adele and meet their specific needs. His criteria were that he could live independently in the first tier and be involved with an active community of his peers and still see Adele as much as possible. For Adele, he wanted a bright and cheerful atmosphere where she could be attended to prudently and safely in the second or third tier, depending on the progression of her Alzheimer's. Although searching for the ideal situation took some time and persistence, Ogden was grateful that he had the time and that the decision was not precipitated by a crisis. On a subsequent visit to Ogden at his new home, I was given the grand tour. Noticeably, Ogden had already made a hit with other residents and staff. Adele was

having lunch in a bright and cheerful dining room with the assistance of an aid. Ogden said he often helps to feed her either lunch or dinner or both. Although he expressed some sadness about the circumstances that led him to make this life change, he had no regrets about the actual choice he had made.

This transition went smoothly for Ogden, mainly because the decision to move to a care facility was made before an actual crisis had taken place. Estelle's experience is in stark contrast. I was surprised when arranging an appointment with her that her speech was somewhat hesitant, and she had given me a new address—St. John's Retirement Villas. On arriving for our visit, I sat down with Estelle in her new little parlor. Her pride and dignity were still apparent in her posture. This stately woman, who deplored dependence and perceived it as a weakness, was now in a retirement facility. I was very curious about what had transpired since our last visit.

Estelle

I knew that my macular degeneration was limiting my ability to take complete care of both Hal and myself, but I wasn't about to give in to it either. I had no intention of giving up our lovely little house in our safe, tree-lined neighborhood in which we'd lived for forty-two years. My daughters, who, as you know, both live out of state, had been encouraging me for some time to move to a facility where I would have less household responsibility and get assistance in caring for Hal. During my older daughter, Rose's, last visit, I begrudgingly agreed to at least look at the facility owned by the church. It's not only been our church for years, but I have some very good friends who live there with whom I regularly play bridge.

About two months after Rose's visit, as I awakened one morning and tried to get out of bed, I had a horrible weakening sensation on the right side of my body and fell to the ground. Luckily I was able to reach the bedside phone and call for help. Even though I made a rapid recovery from the initial trauma caused by the stroke, I was left with some aphasia and a minimal paralysis on my left side, which is improving somewhat with therapy. It was glaringly apparent that I could no longer trust myself to be alone with Hal and responsible for the two of us. So, in the midst of recovery, I sold our home and prepared to move to St. John's. My daughters came, and everyone rallied around us. Friends, neighbors, as well as church members pitched in to help me. Although I balked at first at accepting their generosity, I gave up my foolish pride and was eternally grateful to all of them.

Estelle's formerly held rigid and faulty belief that dependence on others was a weakness to be deplored was altered and reconstructed. Because of this experience, she gained the grace to receive, while maintaining her pride and independence. This change and its positive outcome are important to consider. Often we sabotage possibilities and progress by clinging to old, erroneous-but-familiar beliefs.

Bill

Hazel is really confused. She's pacing all day and is easily agitated. Her doctor gave me some medications to calm her, but I still have to watch her all of the time. She shuffles her feet and just can't pick them up when she walks. As a result, she fell last week and bruised her cheek. Just yesterday she tumbled again, and the whole right side of her body is black and blue. It's all due to this bloody Alzheimer's. If you saw her though, you'd swear that I'd beaten up on her.

I'm thinking more and more that I should place her. But I'm so ambivalent. On my weaker days I feel shame and guilt and I call myself a quitter for not being strong enough to hang in there with her. On my stronger, more rational days I'm keenly aware of the warning signs. She needs more than I can give her.

That was several months before Bill decided to place Hazel. Because he was unable and unwilling to take time for himself, he was exhausted and becoming more isolated and depressed and had frequent bouts of crying. Subsequently, at the caregivers' support group, when it was his turn to unload, Bill spoke quietly, his face grave, his lips taut.

> I placed Hazel a week ago. This was the hardest decision I've ever made in my life. I was so unsettled, consumed with self-judgment and self-pity, and so uncertain of myself. Faltering and straddling the fence is not characteristic of me. Neither was my temper and impatience with Hazel. I have always loved Hazel and yet I found myself no longer treating her lovingly. I wondered whether I had been paying attention to what would be best for her. I realize now that I was obviously exhausted and couldn't look objectively at the big picture. Poor Hazel, what must this have been like for her?
>
> One day—aha! It was like a lightbulb went off in my head. I knew what I had to do, and that was to place Hazel in an Alzheimer's facility, and so I did.
>
> I'm finding in just these few days, that I am more kind, gentle, and affectionate toward Hazel. That's what she needs from me. That is the essence of my role in her life now. Let the professionals at the nursing home provide her with the physical care that she requires. Because she is so oblivious of her surroundings, she seems to have settled down okay. Of course, even though it's been only a few days and I'm still on the roller-coaster ride, I have no doubt that I've made the right decision.

Betty

According to Betty, her marriage to Elliott had never been a happy one. She said that before Alzheimer's he was an aggressive and successful businessman. He was also obnoxious and treated her in a demeaning, unappreciative way, often making her the humiliating brunt of his jokes. Publicly, she hid her resentment and hurt, while privately, she suffered much sadness, internalizing her feelings of distress and alienation toward Elliott.

They were members of one of the private clubs and lived in a large ranch-style home within its security gates. For a long time after Elliott was diagnosed with Alzheimer's, Betty put aside her feelings and committed to taking care of him at home for as long as she could. With the illness, however, he only became more aggressive and mean-spirited. Much to Betty's chagrin, he'd constantly try to get out of the house. Even after she had installed double locks on the doors, Elliott would manage to sneak out, particularly on the days that the housekeeper was there. Elliott would insist that he was going to play golf and would not take "no" for an answer, threatening her with his club when she refused to take him. For fear of her safety, she put him on medication recommended by his physician to calm him. The medication took the edge off the anger, but as the illness progressed, he became more and more difficult to control and fought her attempts to feed, dress, and bathe him. It took a terrible toll on Betty, and eventually, she was forced to give up her role as full-time caregiver.

With the full support of their children, Betty placed Elliott, but within a short period of time, she was consumed with feelings of guilt and ambivalence, questioning her motivation. Did she place him out of anger? Was this betrayal? Was this her way of punishing him? Was she acting out of her own selfishness? If he had been a loving husband, would she have placed him? At one point she even brought him home, thinking she could try taking care of him again. It took a long time, along with the tireless support of her children and friends, for her to absolve herself of guilt about the decision to place Elliott. In the meantime, she sold the house that seemed filled with more bad memories than good and, taking only her favorite treasures, moved into an adult living facility. Much to her delight she soon encountered a number of youthful, spirited seniors like herself and participated in activities that she had previously enjoyed. Eventually, when the facility added a hospital wing specifically for patients with Alzheimer's disease, she moved Elliott there and lived with him on the same campus until the day he died.

Hedda

Even though Hedda placed Abraham in a facility where the staff seemed very caring and competent, she decided she would go there at lunchtime every day to feed him. Her reasoning was that even though the staff were capable, they probably did not have enough time to sit with all the Alzheimer's patients individually and assist them, making sure they were eating adequately. She knew one needed to take a lot of time with Abraham. Here she explains the evolution of the "Faircrest Feeders."

> You know, Mary, before I broke my arm and had to place Abe he wasn't eating well at home. He would chew for a long time and sometimes just seem to forget to keep eating or lose interest. Who knows? Anyway, no matter how caring they are at Faircrest Manor, I wasn't sure they could spend enough time making sure Abe was eating. So I started going there every noon to feed him. What I soon discovered was that there were several of us who would show up at the same time for this same reason. We began to chat with each other as we were feeding our spouses and, over time, became friends. We'd talk about our kids, our marriages, the whole kit and caboodle. Caregiving gave us the commonality that drew us together. Basically, we understood a lot about each other at the outset. Now we sometimes go out for little celebrations. For instance, last week Louie turned seventy and, after feeding our spouses, we all went to lunch. Zeke found

writing poetry was a good outlet for him in the lonely evenings. He'd try out all of his latest on us. Like:

"Washeth"

He who washeth for himself
And puteth dish upon the shelf,
He the Lord will surely bless
For cleaning his unholy mess!

"Outrageous"

There are those who,
In meter Ogden Nashen,
Would try to cash-in
On his style and form, and worse,
Of poetry so perverse,
With convoluted works and phraseous
That twist the mind and tongue
In manners most outrageous.

He is such a hoot. The most unexpected outcome of our friendship is that when one of us isn't able to be there at lunchtime, whether we're ill or taking a vacation to see the kids, one of the other Feeders will make sure our spouse eats. It's made our labor of love much easier. We're really having fun and we've become such good friends.

TRANSITIONING TO LIFE ALONE

As these stories show, ultimately, most caregivers do adjust to this unwanted separation in spite of the loss, although adapting to an absent spouse is easier for some than for others. By now, fairly adept at tapping into your inner resources, you will again find the strength to cope. It's important to be patient with yourself and move through this grieving process at your own pace. After all, these years were meant to be "golden," and many dreams about that future together have been shattered. Allowing time to cry, to be angry, or to be filled with self-pity as well as the whole range of emotions you are experiencing can be very healing. Having the support of family, friends, or a therapist is essential in calming these tumultuous emotions. Joining an Alzheimer's support group to be with others who are dealing with this exact situation can also be very healing. Talking openly about your thoughts and reactions can take the sting out of those burning emotions.

Physical recovery can aid in the emotional healing. Whether you have experienced significant health problems (e.g., high blood pressure, angina, or chronic back pain) before placing your spouse or are merely exhausted, relief is now possible. It's amazing what a good night's sleep, less physical exertion, eating regularly and slowly, or just taking off your shoes and putting your feet up in the middle of the day will do for your health. Getting through the day without being constantly alert to your patient's aberrant behavior lowers the stress level immeasurably. Time again is your friend in regaining your equilibrium, health, and composure.

Darlene

I loved my job as a financial aid officer in the department of admissions at the community college. When Ernie was healthy I would look forward to coming home from work, knowing that over supper with him, I could share my day. Often we would commiserate about a particular student in need of financial aid and share the delight when one of them was able to overcome his hardships and achieve academic success. I really felt I was doing something worthwhile at the college. However, as Ernie needed more care I cut back on my hours at school. Over time his needs became greater and greater. I continued on this treadmill, not really functioning at my best at school or at home. I just kept going. At night I would collapse and hope that Ernie would sleep through the night. This went on for two years.

Three months ago Ernie fell and I just couldn't grab him in time. He suffered a few bruises and tore up his knee. I know this sounds horrible, but it was almost a blessing in disguise. It forced the issue of placing him. I was able to realize then that I was too tired, weak, and run-down to continue taking care of him. I realized that I, too, had to recuperate. This meant no more eating on the run or not eating at all and no more sleep deprivation or broken sleep. I no longer needed to be constantly vigilant to keep Ernie safe from himself. While actively caring for Ernie, I had no idea how draining that alone had been.

Eventually, I began to think about putting the parts of my life together. With less to do at home I was beginning to feel bored and useless. So I called the community college to ask if I could return to work part time. I was nervous about making the call and worried that since I'd been replaced, perhaps there would be no openings. However, my old supervisor said she would be delighted to have me back. This week I've returned to my job at the college. I feel I'm able to give the students my full attention again and make decisions in their best interest. Now when I come home from work I don't have to muster up the energy to start my second job. I do miss sharing my experiences with Ernie very much. He doesn't recognize me anymore, but I visit him every other day, on my short days at work, and usually stay to feed him his supper. I'd give anything to have Ernie whole again, and sometimes I feel terrible when I say good-bye to him in the nursing home, but I know that I really did the best I could in caring for him as long as I possibly could.

It was rewarding and stimulating for Darlene to be back in the workforce. Not only did it reinstate her confidence and self-worth, but it was also a job that gave her a great deal of pleasure. In being forced to take time to heal she was able to put her own vulnerability and human weakness in perspective and regain objectivity as well as a renewed optimism about life once again. This was a triumphant experience for Darlene, who indeed began to reinvent her life.

CHAPTER 16

When Alone Equals Lonely: Loneliness and Companionship

Even while your Alzheimer's spouse is still living at home, like many caregivers, you may have much to say about how lonely your marriage has become. Devoid of conversation, sexual intimacy, recognition, and the rewarding interplay that gave your relationship meaning, you struggle to make sense of what your marriage has become and how you define yourself and this partnership. When your partner no longer recalls who you are or understands the concept of loyalty and fidelity or marriage in general, what happens then? True, you have tied the wedding knot and affirmed the marriage vows that consolidated the conjugal bond. Most of you have remained unwavering in your devotion to your spouse, continuing to provide loving care whether at home or in placement, until death do you part. Nonetheless, we all need to feel a sense of belonging and reciprocity. Caregivers are no different from the rest of mankind, who feel this need intensely. The need for a congenial relationship, to feel loved, to enjoy the company of a friend, and to have a sexual relationship does not diminish with age.

Even those of you who have supportive children and good friends deplore how forsaken and lonely and how irrevocably changed your marriage has become, ravaged by Alzheimer's disease.

In these circumstances not only do most of you continue to cope as best as you can, enhancing your lives with activities outside of your caregiving duties, but some of you might also feel blessed to find a companion who brings new meaning and vitality into your lives.

At one support group meeting, some brave souls talked openly about their views on this awkward, personal, and very sensitive topic. They disclosed their feelings and confusion on the complex and untraditional role of being married but not in the customary and natural sense of the word, and the matter of dating or becoming involved with someone. For many caregivers, whose mean age is seventy, dating, romantic trysts, fraternizing with the opposite sex—while legally married—are threatening topics to discuss.

Nate had attended the support group for four years before he arrived at the point where he felt without question that his only recourse was to place his wife, Flora. He had been a remarkable caregiver. Seeming restless during the group discussion, when it was his turn to talk, he was obviously struggling to find the right words. He scratched his head and looked down for a moment before he spoke in a barely audible voice.

Nate

As you all know, placing Flora was a tough decision for me to make. I wondered whether I had done the right thing, and I even brought her home after she had been in the nursing facility for three months. Once she was home again I realized that I couldn't cope, and back she went to the facility, forcing us to readjust again. My focus has always been on Flora, and often I wondered how I could stand it if I couldn't see her curly head on her pillow next to mine. Now that query is as real as can be. I've been in therapy, which has helped me to grieve and refocus my life a little. Seeing how lonely I am, my cleaning lady often told me that what I needed was a girlfriend. I would laughingly agree with her, like it was a joke. When people have spoken about companions that have helped ease their loneliness, I must admit, I've been skeptical and even judgmental—until it happened to me.

With these preliminary statements out of the way, I want to tell you that about a month ago, I met a lovely widow, Agnes, at the senior center. We chatted some and since then we've had lunch many times and have even gone to a movie or two. She's a delightful companion. We talk as if there's no tomorrow. It's a poignant reminder of how long it's been since Flora and I have had any kind of meaningful conversation. I love my Flora and always will. Agnes knows all about her and that I cannot commit to anything more than a friendship. I almost feel I'm confessing to a bad deed in telling you this. In all truth, I feel some shame and, of course, that ever-present and cunning foe, guilt. I'm worried also about how I'm being judged by you right now. I debated for a while about whether to bring this up but chanced that you have always listened to me with openness and compassion whether or not in complete agreement with me. Being with Agnes has suddenly changed my whole perception and attitude on the subject. Although I was coping with the loneliness, I watched some of you take back parts of your life. Instead of remaining cynical and afraid, I began to step out of my narrow boundaries and leave myself open. I know I've changed in amazing ways over the slow course of Flora's illness and realize that I'm still evolving. Since I've met Agnes, I feel as if I'm at least ten years younger and have a new sense of optimism about my life. I hope I'm not offending you all.

Nate took a deep breath and let it out slowly. He gave an awkward grin, revealing his discomfort, and looked questioningly around the table at his fellow caregivers. No one spoke immediately. This is a very uneasy but significant issue, and no one regarded its consequences as trifling. Then Carolyn broke the silence.

> Gosh, Nate, I've always admired your frankness. I, for one, truly understand what you have just said, and am struggling with the idea—that is, what if I happen to meet someone and would like to encourage a more meaningful friendship? What would I do? You have given me permission to feel more open to that possibility.

Mannie, trying to assuage Nate's guilt, said:

> Because people do take their vows seriously, it is no wonder they feel guilty. However we are not living a normal life, nor do we have a traditional marriage, and we ought to take that into account.

Angela, who was always outspoken and honest about her views, gently spoke to Nate and the group.

> I don't think I would ever be able to be comfortable with another person. It's just not in me. But I wouldn't condemn you or others, who do reach out and become involved with someone else. I really do understand.

Some members of the group remained noticeably silent. Leonard broke the quiet.

Leonard

> I think this is an opportune time for me to put my two cents in. I really understand, buddy. In the group we've used the words "married widows and widowers," and I've identified

with that concept. It's hard not to. This whole confusing issue, which is bound by the morals with which we were all raised, has taken a lot of thought and many a discussion with my family and friends.

More than learning how to take care of Rene, I've learned from all of you the importance of believing that we all deserve a life of quality, and that we must take care of the parts of our lives that still have significance for us. I find that I have, even in my advancing years, been able to develop the capacity to be more open and flexible in my actions, thoughts, and beliefs. Regarding extramarital relationships, I realize that twenty years ago this would have been completely unacceptable in my mind. But times have changed, and we are in a very unique circumstance.

My daughters, much to my surprise, have urged me to find a companion. They worried about me being home alone so much and saw, perhaps more than I, how isolated I had become.

The point is, I, too, have met a really nice gal, Phyllis. Her husband passed on a few years ago. It seems to me that when two lonely people meet, they talk, and both want to get some TLC. As you know, when I placed Rene two years ago, it was devastating to me. I sort of pulled myself up by my bootstraps, but I'd been feeling like a sour old man. Things are different now, since I met Phyllis. I feel young, like a kid again. I don't know how many years I have left, but I'm not dead yet. As a matter of fact, right now I feel very much alive.

I've been forthright with Phyllis. She doesn't intrude on the time I have with my wife. I've introduced her to the girls, who, as I have said, are accepting of this relationship. I refrain from displays of affection between us in front of them. They're not ready for that, and I respect their feelings.

In all honesty, I do feel some shame and some guilt, but at the same time, I try not to care about what other people think. This is my life. I have the choice to live it or to isolate myself and remain lonely and dispirited until I die.

The other night I took my bright red pajamas and a bottle of wine over to Phyllis's. She cooked a delicious meal for us. We chatted and laughed and watched TV. When I woke up in the morning, I was disoriented at first. Then I realized that I was in Phyllis's home, lying on the sofa. I had fallen asleep watching the TV, and Phyllis was kind enough to cover me with a quilt and leave me in dreamland. Is this me? I wondered.

Leonard's eyes sparkled with amusement as he looked around the table at his friends. He nodded his head, and then sat back with the wide and satisfied grin of a Cheshire cat.

Most of the participants teased Leonard, as they often did. Almost all had smiles on their faces. A few looked thoughtful.

Over the years, the core members of the caregiver group had formed a bond and felt safe bringing up their concerns and fears about any issues revolving around their caregiving. In this nonjudgmental, compassionate atmosphere, participants' openness, and their right to their core beliefs, were respected, and each individual's right to privacy was kept sacred. What was shared stayed within the group.

As you might suspect, it is not unusual that members in a group might become attracted to one another. A relationship did evolve between two longtime attendees, Yvette and Bill.

Yvette

Yvette's husband had been placed for about three years, and Bill's wife had died two years earlier. Bill, a great contributor and core member of the group, continued to attend even though his wife was deceased. The group seemed to notice little goings-on with Yvette and Bill. For instance, they were keenly aware that whoever arrived first would save a seat for the other. As time went on, their affection for each other became more obvious. Since Yvette was still married, this relationship was very hard for her to come to terms with. She debated in her own mind about what to do for many anxious months. They were two lonely people. They both enjoyed each other's company very much. Bill made her laugh and feel very worthwhile. Her children approved of their affiliation. There were the moral issues for her of being a married woman and remaining a good Christian. She spoke with a counselor and to her pastor. Bill stood by patiently, allowing her the space and time she needed. Finally, she seemed to make peace with her feelings of guilt and eased into what became a wonderful friendship. In the group, they seemed content, compatible, and visibly happy.

It was important for Yvette to begin to adapt to the life ahead of her. She was very aware of the foreboding and ominous reality that she would soon become a widow. With a propensity toward depression, it was imperative that Yvette develop some hope and optimism for the future and to have compassion for herself and nourish her spirit. She also needed to feel a sense of mastery and control. In her counseling sessions she had found a middle ground that allowed her to accept her new life and give up self-criticism, admonishment, and guilt. There was no question that she would always love her husband and that she would not abandon him. She retained her spiritual connection with God and honored her right to a fulfilling existence.

It's worth repeating that there is no question of your devotion and commitment to your spouse during your caregiving journey. The gift of finding a friend, a companion, to fill the void of loneliness should be looked at maturely and reasonably in the context specific to your situation.

The tumult and intensity of feelings experienced by you and your family in the late-middle stages of Alzheimer's is tremendous. The loss of the "person" in your patient, your relinquishment of the role of primary caregiver, and the succeeding loss of identity and the loneliness that may follow are all monumental outcomes. What we hope we have imparted in this chapter is the means to acknowledge your humanness; to come to terms with intense negative emotions, particularly those of grief, guilt, and loneliness, and to then feel empowered and responsible for maintaining a life rich in relationships and self-fulfillment.

PART FOUR

THE FINAL STAGE AND BEYOND

CHAPTER 17

Nearing the Journey's End: Final Stages of Alzheimer's

Yvette

When I think of my husband in his healthy years, he always seemed larger than life. Rich was strong, robust, and very passionate about his job as a fireman. Over those forty-two years of service, I'd never seen him hesitate when receiving a call, whether to rescue families from a raging apartment fire or a kitten from atop a tree. It was all very gratifying to him. I was so proud of Rich but worried every time I heard the sirens, knowing full well the perils of his job. When he'd come home after his shift I'd usually massage his neck and shoulders, comfort him in times of loss, or celebrate his crew's courageous rescue with him, while silently thanking God that he came home safely.

Richard has had Alzheimer's disease for at least ten years

now, and he's been in a nursing home for almost six. Right now, I would say that he's in the final stage of Alzheimer's disease, as he's completely helpless. He hardly eats and continues to lose weight. He's down to 120 lbs. Much of the time he lies in bed in a fetal position.

When I think about who Rich was at the time we first married and compare that likeness to the visual image I now have, I'm saddened and maddened at the way in which this disease has consumed him.

As he has reached different levels of deterioration, I've slowly said my good-byes to him. When he dies, I want to feel content knowing in my heart that I've told him how much I love him, how I'll miss him, and that I've always known how much he loved me. I want him to know what our marriage has meant to me, how much I've depended on him and admired his strength and kindness. I don't want to leave anything unsaid.

Earlier in the illness we would hold hands, or hug each other and even cry together, but now he doesn't outwardly respond to my touch or my voice, although I do think I see his eyes glistening at times and he sort of moans. It's painful to see him at this stage. I don't go in every day to visit him and haven't for a long time, but I call the nurses daily to get an update on his condition. I'm in limbo, however, up one day and down the next. The whole process of dealing with this illness is that you are always treading water as you struggle to keep up and adapt to the ever-changing stages that this disease presents to you. I am also grieving—this has been a long, long good-bye, with far too many losses.

Now I'm trying a different type of closure. I feel ready to let him go. I'm telling him that he's the leader in the family and that we'll join him later. In this way, I'm letting him know that it's okay for him to let go. I reassure him that we will be all right without him. I couldn't have told Rich this before now. It's taken a while for me to feel really confident in my

> ability to take care of myself. I believe I can do so now; after all, I've been alone for six years. Occasionally, when I've told my friends what I'm doing, and they ask me if he understands, I tell them that I don't know but it doesn't matter. I consider it important for me to do this. In many ways when I say things out loud after mulling them over in my head, it tends to affirm that these ideas are indeed true for me. I know I'll be able to get on with my life until it is time for us to be together again. If he understands what I'm saying and feels comforted by it—all the better.
>
> Thankfully, my children continue to be involved and supportive of my decisions. I get strength from this support group, my friends who have hung in there with me throughout Rich's illness, and also from my strong faith. I figure I'm still walking, talking, and breathing. I have so much to be thankful for.

Yvette pursed her lips and lowered her eyes, her curly gray head nodding slightly. The group members waited for her to continue. When she raised her head, her resolve was obvious to all of us. Yvette grinned, and recalling her initial attendance in the caregiver's support group, she continued.

> I ought to get the award for the most improved caregiver in this group. I know, as most of you do, that I was a basket case when I first came here. I had sunk into a deep depression. I couldn't even say the words "Alzheimer's disease." I can hardly believe it's me telling you how poorly Rich is faring, in an almost unemotional way, and that I'm prepared for it to be over. But I am. This is truly the way I feel. I'm ready to get on with the rest of my life.

Yvette's story, in which she describes Rich's current condition and her coping, and alludes to her rocky emotional history, represents an excellent example of the evolution of a caregiver. Since Yvette was in both the support group and the Caregiver Study, we who have observed her over time can attest to her remarkable renaissance. When we first met, Yvette was very frightened and bewildered. She had a hard time conceiving of how she would handle the next several years, as she not only lacked a sense of self-confidence, but also had been very dependent on Richard and yielded much of the day-to-day responsibility to him. She also had a propensity toward depression. Here, in the final days of her husband's life, she talks with bemused pride about where she is currently—emotionally prepared, stout-hearted, with a sense of well-being and self-worth, and even some optimism for the future. This is also the turning of the tide of her passage through care giving—Yvette has come to terms.

Nate

As Flora's health declined, Nate made every effort to keep the attachment between the two of them alive, even though he was never sure how much she really understood. He had watched with an ache in his heart as she lost the ability to stand up straight, then as she began to shuffle as she walked, tilted to one side, necessitating the use of a walker, and ultimately as she became wheelchair bound. Concurrently, all of Flora's abilities declined. She could no longer feed herself and had to be coaxed to eat. She had lost her ability to speak.

At one of the support group meetings, Nate shared some of his innermost experiences as he watched Flora reach the end stages of Alzheimer's disease. His deep voice faltered, though his gaze was penetrating.

> Throughout Flora's illness and hospitalization, I've been able to show empathy for her as well as for myself. I never would have believed this metamorphosis in my character was possible. Now I regard myself as a nicer, kinder man. In spite of the destructive proclivity that this disease has had on us and

after the rough beginnings as a rather resentful and angry caregiver, I've been able to sustain a gentle and loving relationship with Flora. From the memories that have defined the essence of our fifty-five-year marriage, I've found the strength to create meaning in our relationship in spite of the devastating effect of Alzheimer's.

When Flora could still speak and was somewhat coherent, we'd reminisce about the things we used to do. I felt so close to her when sharing those happy memories. I never knew how much she really understood, but she often laughed at stories I told or nodded her head in agreement or possibly remembrance.

I would also take her on outings. We'd drive around in the car or park at the pier, and I'd play tapes of some of our favorite tunes—"Sunrise, Sunset" and other songs from *Fiddler on the Roof.* We'd hold hands and tears would roll down our cheeks. Those moments were so intimate and tender; I feel that I connected with her in a most profound way in spite of the disease.

As her illness progressed, I'd sit next to Flora's hospital bed, and as I gently caressed her arm, I'd tell her I loved her and would ask her if she loved me. When she could no longer speak, she would whimper and tighten her grasp on my arm. As incognizant of her environment as she seemed, I was amazed at how she still seemed able to react emotionally.

There were times when I'd feel sad and often at some unguarded moment, tears would fill my eyes. I could be anyplace, at the park or watching a program on TV. As difficult as the grieving is, I like that I have those tender feelings. I never thought that I could be so openly gentle and nurturing. In the past, I always recoiled from any outward, gushy displays of affection.

Now I'm wondering, as I'm facing Flora's final days, how I'll cope with her death. I expect that it won't be too well. For one thing I'm still hanging on to all these layers of guilt.

> This statement took the group by surprise and Mannie, Nate's close friend, interrupted. "Nate do you mean after telling us all this, you're still clutching on to guilt?"
>
> Nate replied spontaneously with a sudden grin on his face. "Yes, I'm still only inclined to let go of my old nemesis, guilt, little by little."

Despite the poignancy and sadness of his story, when he made that remark, he and the group burst out laughing, for we all knew of Nate's roller-coaster ride with this battle to conquer guilt. We all appreciated his ability to laugh at himself and his own foibles. The humor in what Nate had said came out of the group members' knowledge of who Nate was, and their longtime association with him. At the beginning of Nate's caregiving, he wrangled with his emotions. The disruptions and unpredictable changes that are part of Alzheimer's disease had caught him off guard and left him feeling confused, angry, resentful, as well as plagued with guilt when he reacted negatively toward Flora. Over time he came to recognize that his behavior was often unreasonable in relation to the incident, and he could laugh when he would catch himself expressing guilt over something minor. Even though the group would try to tease him out of it, they were often perplexed by Nate's capacity for guilt in light of his otherwise extraordinary coping skills.

Nate's successful coping came about once he could sort through the disorderly and negative emotions, find a sense of equilibrium, and experience compassion for both himself and Flora. Now Flora is at the end stage of Alzheimer's, and Nate is somewhat speculative and uncertain about how he will rise to the occasion.

Both Nate and Sylvia's stories are excellent examples of how emotional chaos was the driving force of transformation and extraordinary growth in two caregivers. As you have learned from the onset of your caregiving experience, psychological variations and shifts are as frequent and varied as the changing color of a chameleon. From the time your spouse was first diagnosed, you entered into a different reality, a macrocosm where your marital relationship and lifestyle were reordained and your life would never be the same.

FINAL STAGE BEHAVIORS

It's in these last stages, as the patient is facing death, that you will confront crucial decisions—whether you extend the life of your loved one or allow it to end naturally. This would mean that you acknowledge and accept the significant markers that herald the approach of death.

What do you observe in this last stage? Your spouse will exhibit a definite evanescence of energy, possibly sleeping most of twenty-four hours. He or she will no longer have an appetite or need for fluid. Many patients become stiff and inflexible or immobile, often curled into a fetal position. Because the patient has become completely dependent, he or she will usually require around-the-clock care. Communication may be limited to grunting sounds as speech has diminished. The brain can no longer tell the body what to do.

Ultimately, in this terminal stage, your loved one may fall peacefully into a coma before the actual death occurs.

CHAPTER 18

The Relief of Planning Ahead: Advanced Directives

Gilbert

Pleasant and polite, Gilbert was also a very private man, always cautious about sharing his deep concerns and feelings with the group. It was obvious, however, that he had a deep and abiding love for his wife, Rosa, and observing her decline was very difficult for him.

Early in the course of Rosa's disease, Gilbert made the decision to care for her at home until her death. In the twelve years that she slowly declined, he would reluctantly add outside caretakers and resources to aid him in his unshakable commitment. For some time he managed quite well on his own. However, over time, her behavior became so disruptive and inconsistent that it became harder and harder to keep her entertained at home. He was at the point of pulling out his already thinning hair before he made the decision to send Rosa to day care three days a week.

Gilbert was very close to his sister and brother-in-law, and they would often fly in from New Mexico and stay several weeks to give him both moral and physical support. These visits always boosted his mood and energy level. His sister, Amelia, was a ball of energy and would take over the kitchen, making tamales and other favorite dishes from their childhood; clean the house from top to bottom; and mend every torn sock she could find. She would also attend the support group meetings with Gilbert and, in direct contrast to him, she was very open to discussing everything around Rosa's illness, often to Gilbert's chagrin.

Despite the slow but progressive deterioration in Rosa, and Amelia's outspoken observations, Gilbert never quite accepted that his wife was as advanced in the illness as she was. He remained hopeful and optimistic and overlooked ominous signs that forewarned of the terminal decline that to many was so visible in Rosa. Alternatively, another conceivable reason for his naked optimism was his unconscious use of denial. He simply was not ready to concede to the damage the disease had wreaked on his wife. Quite out of character, one day in the group he poured out his story.

> Rosa was pretty advanced in the Alzheimer's when she had a sudden TIA—a ministroke. I kept her home from day care for a few weeks, and when she seemed strong enough to return, I started her back in the program. She was a little slower and more confused, but it wasn't enough to concern me. She liked attending the day-care program, and I was really happy with the care and attention she received over there.
>
> I was feeling somewhat comfortable again when *Ka-pow-ee* another disaster caught me completely off guard. Be forewarned. There's a lesson in this for all of us. I'm here to tell you that no one can ever rest peacefully or fool themselves into thinking there's any predictability when dealing with this damned Alzheimer's.
>
> One day, while at day care, Rosa fell backward in her chair, hitting the floor. The director immediately called me,

and I rushed out to meet her and Rosa at the hospital. The doctor's initial evaluation was that nothing horrible had happened, but since Rosa seemed to be under the weather and in some pain, I decided to keep her home the next day. Late that afternoon, the doctor called to tell me that Rosa had actually broken a bone in her neck. She was admitted to the hospital with twenty-four-hour care. I didn't realize it then, but Rosa would never return home again.

My determination to keep her at home was defeated not by the effects of Alzheimer's disease but by an unpredictable accident. From that point on, Rosa rapidly deteriorated. She wouldn't eat. In no time at all she lost thirty pounds. I was beside myself. My sister and brother-in-law flew in to be with me. Their support was a godsend.

Rosa's doctor, along with the hospice nurses, concurred that Rosa was showing the signs of approaching death. Now I had to make the big decision. Do I put her on tube feeding to keep her alive? Alzheimer's may be winning, but I still held the trump card. That is until it struck me that long before Rosa even got Alzheimer's she had signed Advanced Directives allowing that no extraordinary means be used to keep her alive. How many times had we discussed this very subject in the group? Yet, I never realized how difficult it would be to follow in the here and now.

I called the hospice nurse, as I wanted to know what Rosa was probably experiencing at this time. The nurse described what happens to the body when a person begins to die. I was so concerned that Rosa would be in pain, or starving or thirsty. I didn't want to deprive her of anything. The nurse reassured me that Rosa was not in pain and she was not hungry. Rosa was letting go of life in a normal way. It was painful to hear this, but the explanation helped me to carry out Rosa's decision.

It seemed that at first, rather than focusing on the painful reality that Rosa was preparing to die, all I could think of was that I was losing Rosa, and I felt out of control. I was impotent. I wanted to hang on to her and save her somehow. The paradox is that as I watched her slipping away, she seemed so peaceful compared to the utter chaos I was experiencing. I decided not to put her on the feeding tube. Four days later my Rosa died.

I can now admit that I was kidding myself when I stubbornly believed that she was doing okay. She never came back as strong as I imagined she had. I fooled myself a whole lot about how much control I really had over any of this, too.

The doctors have listed Alzheimer's disease as the cause of death, but I won't really know for sure. Since we don't have children, I've chosen not to have Rosa's brain autopsied. If we did have kids, I would have wanted that definitive diagnosis for their sake.

My plans for the future are up in the air. I'm going to go to New Mexico for a few weeks and then we'll see. If I find it's too tough to go it alone, I'll sell the house here and return to New Mexico, where I've got Amelia and the rest of the family.

In an unselfish and loving way, Gilbert did all that he could for Rosa, even to the end in allowing her a natural death. Feeling sure of this in retrospect and acknowledging how resourceful he had been gave him a sense of peace and the ability to move on with the rest of his life.

ALLOWING FOR A NATURAL DEATH

We would like to talk a little bit about what happens to the body when life-sustaining treatment is not implemented. Your doctor and hospice nurses are experts in monitoring and providing optimal comfort to your patient. They can also offer specific information to you and your family so that you will understand the physiology of what is taking place as one's body dies. When you decide to forego giving antibiotics, cardiopulmonary resuscitation, hydration, and nutrition to your spouse, this means you will be giving permission to hospice and medical personnel to allow your spouse's body to undergo the process of naturally shutting down. Using palliative care only, which means that medical intervention is based solely on the comfort of the patient, is highly recommended by most primary care physicians of patients with Alzheimer's disease. Death is increasingly recognized as an integral and important stage of life.

The following is a brief overview of what happens to the body in varying degrees and at different times in the final days of life.

The signs and symptoms can be complex and disorderly. Some time before your patient approaches death in the final stages of Alzheimer's, eating becomes more challenging. Remembering how to chew and how to swallow becomes difficult and eventually impossible, way beyond the patient's abilities. When chewing becomes untenable, your patient will usually be switched from solids to a soft diet until swallowing even puréed food becomes beyond possibility. Eventually your patient will cease to have any appetite.

In the mid- to final stages, you may also find that it has become an effort for you to get an adequate amount of fluids into your spouse, and may worry that dehydration can present even more problems. However, during the dying process, even giving liquids interferes with the body's natural shutting down. It appears that dehydration, as it occurs in the last few days of life, often relieves end-stage symptoms and contributes to a diminished, quiescent level of consciousness. It is an automatic and normal state that occurs when we die. As our body shuts down, individual organs, such as the kidneys, can no longer do the work they were designed to do. It requires a great deal of energy for your patient to consume and digest even water. It is the general consensus of hospice that patients are often more comfortable and relieved of suffering end-stage symptoms if dehydration is permitted rather than forcing fluids. The cessation of fluids can also eliminate the need for a Foley catheter, which is used to drain fluid from the bladder, or a nasogastric suction tube used to relieve pressure caused by excess fluid in the stomach. Pain medications are frequently unnecessary at this point, and the patient is allowed to drop into a coma. The burden of even a simple IV may exceed its benefits and cause acute discomfort. Reduced fluids and increased electrolytes serve almost as natural anesthesia for the central nervous system, because the patient's level of consciousness diminishes and his or her perception or sensation of suffering decreases. The patient is also monitored for fluid retention in the lungs as well as edema. The most discomforting consequence of dwindling body fluid is usually dry mouth and lips. However, regularly swabbing your patient's mouth with lemon-flavored glycerin swabs and applying lip emollients or Vaseline will help to reduce or alleviate that problem.

If your spouse has been on prescribed medications, they may no longer be necessary at this time. Because of the decreased food and fluid intake, continuing some medications—for example, a blood pressure medication—could actually be harmful. However, your physician may recommend a pain medication such as morphine or an opiate derivative. Pain medications can be given sublingually (under the tongue), rectally, or as a skin patch. Your spouse's physician should carefully monitor all medications. The goal is to keep your spouse comfortable and as pain-free as possible.

Again, we stress that you should question the doctor and hospice personnel so that you are fully educated about this process in reference specifically to your loved one. This will allow you to act knowledgeably and with your loved one's best interest in mind. It will also be reassuring for you to know all that you can.

We are aware of the emotional turmoil you may have around the subject of the dying process, and that it may be difficult for you to read through what we have just written. We are presenting you with all of this information to help eliminate some angst or confusion over allowing dehydration or the natural shutting down of the patient's body to take place, and to emphasize that this natural process allows for an ultimately compassionate and comfortable death for your loved one.

CHAPTER 19

Another Paradox: Anticipatory Grief and Mourning

Lars

Six years ago, because of his own debilitating health conditions, Lars had been forced to place Helga. He had had open-heart surgery and was also a diabetic with some neuropathy in his feet.

He went to see his wife daily, and for a long time, at each visit he would present her with a sweet treat, usually chocolate, which was her favorite. Helga was as delighted as a child and would savor every bite. One day, she rejected the treat and responded to him as if he were a total stranger. To him it was a shift that seemed unbearable, and his emotions were in a tailspin. That occurred many months ago.

> Helga hasn't recognized who I am for a long time. She's no longer able to eat even puréed food. She's been fading away before my very eyes. Last weekend, the nursing home put her

> on hospice, as she has developed pneumonia. At that time, I confirmed with them our decision in the Advanced Directives that Helga receive no extraordinary measures, which at this point would mean not giving her antibiotics.
>
> I'm in limbo—I don't know what I'm doing. One day I feel up, and the next I'm down. Some days I don't want to go and see Helga, and other times I do. I wake up every morning keenly aware that I have not yet received that dreadful, anticipated phone call. During the day, when the phone rings, I think, "That's it, that's got to be the call." I'm trying to prepare myself for the inevitable by practicing, rehearsing if you will, and pretending each day, that when I wake up I'll find out that Helga is no longer alive. I'm doing this so that when she does actually go, it won't be so hard on me. I say over and over again to myself that I know Helga would be better off dead, but I'm having difficulty trying to prepare my heart for that final good-bye. I'm so tired of this damned disease. Can I say, "I wish it were over"?

How do we understand the dynamics of anticipatory grief? Therese Rando, in *Clinical Dimensions of Anticipatory Mourning*, defines it as, "the phenomenon encompassing the processes of mourning, coping, interaction, planning, and psychosocial reorganization that are stimulated and begun in part in response to the awareness of the impending loss of a loved one and the recognition of associated losses in the past, present, and future."

Anticipatory mourning is a clear expression of the paradox of this book—staying connected while letting go. You will find, as you observe your loved one decline and face the threat of his or her impending death, that you wish to hold on to and remain close to him or her while you also struggle to let go. What a dilemma! In essence, although your loved one is alive and facing death, you respond with anxiety and grieving as you anticipate the final permanent separation. The intensity of your reaction coincides with how central and meaningful this relationship has been to you in your life. It is of primary importance that you maintain a balance amid your conflicting emotions, such as love and hate, joy and sadness, frustration and relief. You can do this by paying attention to your thoughts in order to recognize where your feelings are coming from. Say to yourself, "It's okay to feel this way." Accept both your feelings and your thoughts without judgment.

Mourning is about how you deal with losses, and incorporated within mourning are all your responses and reactions to grief. As you mourn and adopt different coping strategies, you will learn that it is these skills that eventually transform you and alter your perception of yourself. You will be amazed to discover that you've grown, matured, and lived through crisis after crisis and survived!

CHAPTER 20

At Peace, My Love: Death of a Spouse

Angela

Angela's husband, Joe, even though declining rapidly for the last several months, had had Alzheimer's for twenty years. Angela cared for Joe at home for almost the entire time. Eventually, he was placed in a care facility, and shortly thereafter, his doctor had requested that he be placed under the care of hospice. Then Joe fell and broke his hip and needed immediate surgery, which seemed to be successful. Angela was expecting that Joe would get through this crisis fairly smoothly and in a timely way. After all, he was gaining strength and walking a little more each day. However, this trauma hastened Joe's decline, and after a few weeks he died. It's not unusual for an Alzheimer's patient who has had a traumatic experience, for example, a fall or surgery, to deteriorate rather quickly.

Angela, always candid and passionate in her commentaries, shared with the group her experience with Joe's dying. Present at the group, just ten days after her beloved husband's death, her face weary and lined with sadness, she recounted the details of those final weeks with Joe.

> At the moment I feel far removed from Joe's death. I haven't cried much. I know I'm grieving. It's different now, and I'm still in shock. I can tell you this, however, and it may sound strange, but Joe's greatest gift to me was in the way he died. I'll come back to that.
>
> It was a hellish three weeks after Joe's fall. At first I fully expected he'd recover, because he was beginning to walk with help. However, two weeks afterward, he began to refuse food and water. He couldn't swallow. His brain hardly seemed to be functioning. The nurses and I agreed that it was dangerous to keep feeding him, as we were afraid that he might choke and food would get into his lungs. He'd already been suctioned once. As you know, Joe and I had very strong opinions about heroics at the end of life, and we had discussions on this very topic many times when he was still mindful and alert. He had been emphatic about having no extraordinary measures taken at the end of his life. During the course of his illness, he'd sometimes cry out to me in agony, "I wish I could die." In compliance with Joe's wishes, he was no longer forced to eat. Prior to this, Joe had been very agitated, but when he stopped eating he was noticeably calmer. One of our daughters, Julie, had come home as soon as she learned of the situation. She wanted to be with both of us at this time. Julie and I were aligned in our approach to Joe's passing, and our hearts were both heavy and light—heavy with the knowledge that he would not be with us in physical form any longer and light because we knew that he was going to feel happy once again. So we released him. We told him how much we loved him and assured him that it was okay for him to go, for we would be just fine. Of course, we were sobbing and holding him and each other.

I must share a light moment Julie and I experienced a few days before Joe died. Here we were, thinking that he was really out of it. We had been in his room with him constantly for two days. A nurse came in to clean him as he had had diarrhea for a few days. As she began to bathe him, we were all startled when we heard his voice as plain as could be. "Uh, uh, uh," he said, "nobody but my wife touches me there." We all three looked at each other, mouths gaping, and then we laughed so hard and for so long. Joe had provided the comic relief we needed at that moment. Dear Joe, his humor never quit to the very end.

Either Julie or I was at Joe's bedside all of the time. We would hold his hand and stroke his arm or talk to him softly. We both felt very much a part of his dying. We also spent a lot of time crying. To pass the time, I would play solitaire on the bed. Every now and then I would become immersed in the game and then suddenly realize I had not checked on Joe. I'd jump up to determine whether or not he was still breathing. He was so still, so quiet. It was important to me to hold his hand, to have some physical connection. Sometimes I'd put down the cards and sit and watch his breathing. The room seemed so tranquil. Even the nurses noticed the serene atmosphere and remarked on how peaceful it seemed.

We reassured Joe over and over again that we would be fine and that it was time for him to go. And on the third day he did. He took a deep breath in and let it out and that was it. We sat with him in the silence for what seemed like a long while before we called the nurse. We felt blessed that we could be with him to the very end. It was a comfort to all of us—to be together.

I have, throughout this disease, told Joe how much I love him. I've hugged him and held him and told him just how wonderful our relationship has been. We did have closure. I feel complete in that I can't think of anything I wish I had said or done for him.

> The nurses gently asked us to leave the room while they prepared his body. We sat in the hallway, numb and exhausted, and I must admit I even felt somewhat elated. A heavy burden had been lifted.
>
> When we reentered the room, the nurses had closed his eyes—well they had attempted to. When I looked at him, his one eye had not quite shut, and he looked as if he was winking at me. My heart skipped a beat and I smiled. How like Joe, I thought.

The group members were still for a moment. Then several spoke at once, offering their condolences to Angela and her family.

> Sylvia said, "Angela, I appreciate your sharing this with us. I often wonder how it will be when Phil dies and sometimes it seems terrifying. I hope that my Phil goes as peacefully."
>
> Bill nodded and made the sign of the cross. "Strange to say, but your story brought me joy and empathy for the experiences you went through. My sympathies to you."

Angela has continued to attend the support group. As a longtime member with a unique understanding of the emotional effects this illness has on the caregiver, her status in the group has changed from member to cofacilitator. As of this writing, two years after Joe's death, she continues to support, love, and listen to the many caregivers who attend the meetings and is a wise, compassionate, and resourceful coleader. Recounting her ordeals and how she was able to prevail has often given hope and alleviated the fear of the unknown for the caregivers attending the group. Most importantly, she lets the other caregivers know that there is help and support out there and that they are not alone.

In advance of Joe's death, Angela had also decided to have his brain autopsied before his cremation. It's necessary to make these arrangements, if this is your desire, well before the death of your patient. This final, practical step in the long course of Alzheimer's disease is important not only for substantiating the diagnosis and cause of death but also because of the genetic implications for the patient's progeny. Within twenty-four hours of Joe's death, the University of California at San Diego Alzheimer's Disease Research Center collected his body so that they could begin to perform the tests that would prove definitively whether or not Joe had had Alzheimer's disease. Within six months Angela received confirmation in the mail from the Department of Pathology and Neurosciences that Joe had indeed suffered from severe and advanced Alzheimer's disease. His brain contained the senile plaques and neurofibrillary tangles of Alzheimer's disease. In addition, the testing revealed that Joe had also suffered two small strokes at some point during his long illness.

Nate

Nate's blue eyes were deep with sadness as he told of his beloved wife, Flora's, death. Through occasional tears and with his voice breaking up at times, he shared his experience with us.

> It's been a while since I attended the group. I was so caught up with Flora toward the end. With the help of hospice, to whom I will be forever grateful, I did everything I could to make her last days on this earth tranquil.
>
> For many months Flora had been not only disinterested in food but also actually unable to eat. For a while she was given fortified drinks, until those coughing spells came on. She got so that when she was fed the drinks through a straw, she would choke and cough for at least thirty minutes to an hour. It was awful to watch. I asked the nurses to try and feed her with a spoon but that was no better. We struggled for a week or so with that. Then I began to ask myself, "What am I doing? Who am I doing this for?" In all honesty, I had to admit that I was trying to save her for me. I wasn't thinking

primarily of her. Bottom line was, I didn't want to see her go. Yet at the same time, I hated seeing her suffer so much.

I'll tell you what I do when I'm facing a dilemma, and you may think that I'm nutty, but it works like a charm for me. I talk things out with myself in the mirror. My therapist suggested that I do this. So I brought my barstool into the bathroom, sat down on it, and looked myself straight in the eye. I said to myself, "Flora has lost so much weight. She is suffering. She'd have wanted to go a long time ago." I felt like an executioner, but the pull to let Flora go was very strong. I decided that that would be my direction and that this was not about me. It was solely about Flora, and I was the only one who could help her at this time.

But to the end, I was still struggling with the paradox—how to stay connected while letting go.

I called both of my sons to get their input. They were both understanding; however, my younger son, desperate to save his mom, suggested we think about tube feeding. It's funny—normally I'd have become impatient and irritated. But I remained calm, realizing the intensity of his feelings and the gravity of our decision. I gently told him to do what I had done—to talk to himself in the mirror. To ask himself the same questions I had asked myself. "What would she have wanted?" He did this, and to my surprise he called a few days later to thank me and said he would support the decision to let his mother die. I hung up the phone with a heavy heart, knowing how difficult it was for my younger son, the apple of his mother's eye, to come to this decision.

In order to reassure myself, I spoke to the hospice nurse about our decision and my fear of Flora suffering if we stopped feeding her and giving her fluids. The nurse explained to me that Flora would not be in pain or suffering, and they would be very attentive to any change as it occurred with Flora. With this knowledge, I told hospice to stop everything.

> Flora lived for about five days without food or water. Her breath became shallow, and she was clearly not in any pain. As I watched her I realized that I was not her executioner. I was allowing her to go peacefully and calmly from this world and the terrible curse of Alzheimer's disease.

Nate paused for a moment and took a deep breath. The frown on his forehead disappeared. His gaze softened and he almost whispered.

> I saw her at peace and I felt so much better. When her breathing became increasingly shallow, I had a cot set up next to her bed and decided to stay with her through the night. I couldn't sleep. I talked to her the whole time. I told her that I was ready to let her go until our spirits would meet again.
>
> In the early morning, my loving Flora died—so peacefully. I was glad that I was with her at the very end. I had heard that with Alzheimer's patients their hearing is the last to go, so I hope she heard the things I said to her. I remember taking a deep breath shortly after realizing Flora was dead and saying to myself, "She's thankful that I let her go." Then I cried and just sobbed. As bereft as I was, I also had a certain peace that is hard to explain. I called my sons and both of them seemed to share the feelings I had. We all knew that she was now in a better place.
>
> It's been a long haul. It was only after at least five years of her behavior becoming increasingly confusing that I even had Flora diagnosed, and that must have been seven years ago. I know I did the best I could for her, and I have come a long way. I've learned to be more compassionate and less self-centered. I've also released a lot of the guilt about Flora having this disease and the way I treated her.
>
> I didn't have a funeral for Flora. Her body was immediately transported to UCSD Alzheimer's Research Center so that we could have her brain autopsied, and then we had

her cremated. We had a small family gathering, which included a memorial service at sea, where, in accordance with her wishes, we dispersed her ashes. The ceremony was wonderful closure for all of us.

By the way, we had discussed the details and arranged for all of these "end of life" decisions many years ago. I hope you have all done this also. It was a great relief to know that we were doing what Flora wished and that prearrangements were in place.

Somehow, I don't feel depressed. I know that I'm continuing to grieve, my heart feels heavy, and yet it also feels light. I know we'll be okay.

The group members had been sitting silently while Nate told his entire story, but they were with him all the way. He knew that. Being a participant in the support group, these were his allies who accepted him, his trials, and his shortcomings with deep understanding and compassion. They knew so well where he was coming from.

Mamie

When I called Mamie to arrange for our six-month interview, she informed me that Bud had died the month before. I anticipated that this visit might be difficult, as Mamie had been intensely committed to Bud's care and loved him dearly. While driving to her home I recalled what a ball of fire this petite women in her seventies was. When I first met her, she was still working part time at a department store and would return home to take on Bud's care, the homemaking, and the gardening. Ruing her own fragile health—she had emphysema and hypertension—she assumed Bud's total care for a long time, until her children and doctor convinced her that she needed to stop.

Mamie would tell me how much strength she derived from knowing that Bud had such an abiding love for her all the years of their marriage. He would often tell her that he didn't deserve her, and she said he treated her like she was a queen. Until the final stages of Alzheimer's, Bud always let her know how appreciative of her he was for everything she did for him. It broke her heart to see the disease take his strength, his pride, and his dignity.

Mamie had to place Bud in an Alzheimer's unit about eight months ago. She went to the nursing home every morning and left right before dark. Everyone on the floor—staff, visitors, and patients—knew her and appreciated her cheerful, engaging presence. While there, she helped with Bud's meals, monitored his enuresis, and talked to him off and on all day. While he slept she visited everyone, read magazines, clipped coupons, or dozed in the chair.

As I stood on the front porch of Mamie's townhouse and she opened the door, I saw immediately that she looked rested, and she smiled broadly, warmly greeting me. In answer to my question, "How are you?" her story began.

> Mary, I'm really all right. Forgive the mess with all these carpet and drapery samples but I'm getting ready to redecorate. You know, I moved to this townhouse to be close to my daughter, Diana, right after Bud was placed and never even had the time to unpack all of the boxes. I've got all of these ideas for changing this dull old place. Everything is going to be teal and pink.

As she looked at the mound of framed photographs on her table, I saw a brush of sadness and melancholy transform her face. Resting on top of the pile was a pastel-painted wedding photo. In a very soft voice, Mamie continued.

> My Bud left me the way I hoped he would. In the last few months there wasn't much left of him. He'd still squeeze my hand and mumble now and then, letting me think that he knew I was there. The last day, the nurses told me he probably wouldn't last much longer. I said I wanted to arrange to

> stay the night, but the nurses said there really was no need. You know, I never stopped talking to Bud, and before I left, I told him I'd be there in the morning and kissed his forehead. He looked right at me, Mary, and I swear he said, "love you." At around 3 A.M., the night nurse, Julia, called to tell me Bud passed away quietly in his sleep.

When I left Mamie after our interview, I recalled that photograph on the table; Mamie looking young and vibrant in her pink suit with matching hat, carrying a small bouquet of white roses, and Bud so handsome and elegant in his army dress uniform. Caught in each other's eyes, these young lovers looked so happy and filled with hope that even with the war on, their love would last forever. "Could it be that Bud really said 'love you'?" I thought skeptically. But I guess it doesn't really matter what my reality was, and besides, who am I to say any different? The importance was the richness and constancy of the love they shared through the evolution of their marriage, even with the intrusion of Alzheimer's disease. Although Mamie by nature was tenacious and determined, the mutual love she and Bud had inspired her caregiving and gave it more sustainable purpose.

CHAPTER 21

Cleaning Out the Closets: the Process of Closure

Cleaning out the closets once your spouse has been permanently placed or is deceased has posed a dilemma for many caregivers. The task is a very personal one and, for many, painful and arduous and leads to some measure of resistance. These material possessions—clothing, jewelry, cards, and photos—are symbols of the history of your unique bond. Recollections of outfits worn for work or special occasions, mementos, keepsakes, and trophies can be, for some, bittersweet remembrances or a caveat to what was the essence of your relationship.

Several of you have shared with us the ways that you have dealt with this task. For some, the preference was to go through these personal belongings in solitude, while for others it was easier to share the experience with family, sorting through everything together, dividing up the more sentimental items and then selling or donating the remainder. Others postponed the task for months or even years.

Mannie

I wasn't sure what to do with my wife's stuff after she was placed, it made me sad to see all her lovely clothes and jewelry lying there, never to be worn by her again. I asked my son and daughter to help me decide what to do. So together we sorted through everything. It was very trying and tiring emotionally and physically for all of us, and we realized there was a lot more stuff to go through than we initially thought. However, we laughed and cried together through the whole lot. My children took what they wanted. I was glad that my daughter wanted the emerald earrings that I'd given Rachel on our first anniversary. One day she'll also have her mother's wedding ring, but Rachel's still wearing it. We put the rest of Rachel's belongings in bags and had them picked up and taken away. I know Rachel would feel good about some needy person enjoying her good dresses and warm coats. Although the experience was disheartening at the time, it was also a relief. I actually felt less burdened once we had completed the job. Having my children there to help was wonderfully comforting for all of us.

Jane said, "I have donated all of my husband's clothing except for his socks. I find comfort in wearing them to bed at night."

"I understand," said Carolyn. "That's why, as you can see, I always wear John's watch."

Bill added, "I've gotten rid of almost everything, except my wife had a drawer full of stuff—nothing of value really. Little trinkets and odds and ends from trips and some cards she'd received that held special meaning for her. I haven't tossed any of those mementos, and I doubt that I will."

"For the last two years, getting rid of, or really letting go of, Phil's worldly goods has simply been too much for me," sighed Sylvia. "I've left everything in his half of the closet and his drawers. Every now and then I'll open the drawer and touch his clothing, then I cry and get on with my day. My kids have tried to get me to part with his stuff. I think I'm almost ready and, when I am, they're willing to help. I've asked them to let me be for now."

"My husband Joe had a very small book in his desk drawer that we'd often chuckle over. It was called *What Men Know about Women*. When you'd turn the page, each page would be blank. It reminds me of his wonderful sense of humor, so I'll keep it forever," declared Angela.

Imelda

Imelda's husband had been placed for over two years and had declined significantly. Her daughters would beg for her to take a break and come to visit them in San Francisco. However, both of them were unwilling to make the trip to San Diego to visit her. Even though their excuses centered around careers, lack of time, or unavailable pet care, she realized they were both reluctant to see their father, as they had yet to come to terms with his illness, especially the younger daughter, Rita.

Imelda felt it was time to give up their large house, which had much more space than she needed and which made her feel all the more lonely. She finally told the girls that she was planning to sell the house and told them they needed to come and visit so that they could take anything they wanted to keep. Rita decided to come down and "get it over with," as she put it. During my visit to Imelda's, she told me what had transpired on the last weekend.

Rita got much more than she bargained for when she came home to go through her old childhood things and to help me with her dad's possessions. Seeing Carlos was really difficult for her. After all, he had been the symbol of strength and competence to her all her life, and she loved him terribly. Sometimes the two of them seemed closer than Rita and I were. They seemed to have a lot in common. Rita was really good at sports and also inherited her dad's gift for music. They both played the guitar. I would often intrude on them in the noisy den and find them dancing together even when Rita was a teenager. How many times did I say, "Carlos! Rita! Turn down that music." Now it's too quiet.

Anyway, Rita seemed to be holding up pretty well until the afternoon of the day before she left. I heard some of the old music coming from the den so I quietly walked in and found her sitting on the floor, amidst all the phonograph records, crying so hard. Mi Hija! It seemed that all of her grief had surfaced with the sounds of the music. I took her in my arms, and we cried together for a long while. She was in such pain, but I felt at the time that she was finally able to release some of her grief.

She left the next day exhausted but feeling very glad that she had decided to finally come down. She's so strong, that one. I know she'll be all right and better now than when she first came. By the way, I went into the den later that day and found a note: "I took some of the records. Thanks Mom. Thanks Dad. Love always, Rita."

Though each caregiver's approach to cleaning out the closet is different, the task universally stirs up many mixed emotions. That's okay. Parting with and reminiscing about your loved one's personal belongings is another way of releasing the past and opening space toward a new future. It should be accomplished in whatever way that you choose.

CHAPTER 22

Honoring Your Tomorrows: Reentry Post Caregiving

We marvel at those of you who, after being separated from your spouse either by placement in a nursing home or by death, are able to reclaim the forfeited parts of your lives. With intense human resolve, you have been able to steadily transition through what has possibly been one of the greatest challenges in your lifetime and move forward to the next stage in your life's journey. Although Viktor Frankl, in his acclaimed book *Man's Search for Meaning,* spoke of a far different type of challenging circumstance, the following quote seems quite fitting, as it is encouraging and entices us to take the steps to make our lives more significant. He states, "Even the helpless victim of a hopeless situation, facing a fate he cannot change, may rise above himself, may grow beyond himself and by so doing change himself. He may turn a personal tragedy into a triumph." Frankl reasons with his reader to "make the best of any given situation." He continues, " . . . the reason I speak of a tragic optimism, that is, an optimism in the face of tragedy and in the view of the human potential which at best always allows for 1) turning suffering into a human achievement and accomplishment; 2) deriving from guilt the opportunity to change oneself for the better; and 3) deriving from life's transistories is an incentive to take responsible action."

In her book *The Places that Scare You,* Pema Chodron, an American Buddhist monk, informs us that we have a choice. "We can let the circumstances of our lives harden us and make us increasingly resentful and afraid, or we can let them soften us and make us kinder."

As you slowly adjust to a new status and begin to recreate your life, one of the discoveries you come to is that your commitment of time and energy in managing the care of your spouse has slowly eliminated a social life that once was very satisfying. It's important to take the steps to reinvolve yourself in the activities and friendships that held meaning for you before you became a caregiver. You will be entering this stage of your life having grown tremendously and having acquired new competencies that will enhance all of the choices you will make.

The following are stories from caregivers who have transitioned to this new status. These brave souls have deliberately started the ball rolling, gathering momentum as they re-create their lives. You have met some of them throughout this book. Here are some examples of how life goes on.

Mannie

Rachel had been deceased for four years at the time of this writing. Mannie had continued to attend the support group for a long while after her death. Then he gradually sat in on the group meetings less and less. It was difficult for him to hear the stories of other caregivers' spouses with Alzheimer's disease. Too close to home, the stories would rekindle old memories or other associations with Rachel. When he was present, though, he still liked to offer suggestions that might be helpful to others.

I interviewed Mannie by phone to inquire about how his life was progressing. We had a lovely conversation at this time. Mannie was warm, friendly, and wonderfully optimistic and positive about his life. Mannie is eighty-nine years young.

The first three years after Rachel died were difficult for me. I came to the support group for a while. It was hard not to after attending for so many years, because we felt like family. Everyone was always so kind and understanding. After a while I felt I needed to move on. I did try a bereavement support group, but after attending it twice, I decided this was not for me. People cried a lot and I felt too much pain. I was depressed during the first three years after Rachel's death, and my doctor prescribed an antidepressant for me that was most helpful. I'm ready to quit taking it now, I'm glad to tell you.

After Rachel died, I left the house as it was, and because we have a lot of photos on the wall, whenever I looked at Rachel or passed by the pictures, I cried. You know, we were married for sixty-five years. We were eighteen years old when we tied the knot. It was during the Depression and we had a hard life at first. Then things improved, and before we knew it, we were contentedly growing old together. However, the last ten years of our marriage, Alzheimer's disease took Rachel and so much of our happiness away from me.

I don't know where I'd be today if it weren't for the support group. You all helped me so much. I remember how helpful it was to me when you told me how concerned you were about the way I looked. Do you remember that? It was at the time when Rachel was incontinent and I was hardly sleeping because she'd be wet, the bed would be soaked, and I had to take care of business. One particularly difficult night it struck me—I said to myself, "It's either her or me. If I die"—and by the way, I was concerned that I might because of my heart condition—"who will take care of Rachel?" I realized that she would end up in a nursing facility, because we had told our daughters that we did not want to be a burden to them. I placed her the next day—it was not an easy thing to do, but I know it was the right thing.

It's taken a while but now I can tell you that I love life. I enjoy it. I like to laugh and have fun. I don't care to focus on

> upsetting or depressing issues. No, I keep my spirits up, and I don't let myself go. People generally don't like to listen to other people's problems, so I don't complain. When people ask me how I'm doing, I ask them, "If I tell you my troubles, can you help me?" They usually respond with a big no, and I tell them, "Okay, so then I won't tell you my problems."

You could hear the titter and amusement in his voice.

> I want to get to one hundred years old and still be in good health. So I take care of myself. I had hip surgery almost a year ago, and little by little I'm getting back into shape. I force myself. I go to rehab three times a week, walk on the treadmill for ten to fifteen minutes, and then ride the bike for thirty minutes.
>
> I have a lovely companion. We've been together for a year now, but I've known her for seven. She lives four doors down from me. She's eight-four and looks good. Her husband also had Alzheimer's and she used to come to the support group meetings that I ran for the members in our residential community. I have no interest in remarrying and neither does my friend. We're very compatible but she's nothing like my Rachel.

I asked Mannie if, while he was caregiving, he ever thought he would feel so happy and content with life again. He told me that he was so sad at that time he couldn't imagine it. His words to me before we said good-bye were, "I want to laugh and have fun. When I die, I want to die laughing and I want to be happy." Happiness did not fall into Mannie's life. In his characteristically deliberate and intentional mind-set, he conscientiously worked to be in a happy state. There is a saying from the Buddha that reminds me of Mannie, "Now may every living thing, young or old, weak or strong, living near or far, known or unknown, living or departed or yet unborn, may every living thing be full of bliss."

Nate

Nate, Mannie's close friend and accomplice throughout his caregiving, shared this story with me by phone six months after Flora passed away. He was open to talking about how he was handling his life after all those years of caregiving. It sounded to me like he had explored this area in depth and felt at peace with where he was now.

He started to tell me about the memorial service that was held at sea.

> With me at the service were my sons, my grandchildren, and Zena, Flora's main caretaker for many years. It was a beautiful service, and at the end, everyone took a handful of ashes and said what they thought or felt in their hearts about Flora. I did okay until the end, when I said, "I love you, sweetheart." I never expected to become so emotional. It was quite an experience for me. I also told Flora, "I know you're looking at us from up there and saying 'Thank you for letting me go and freeing my spirit. I'm very grateful.'"
>
> Sometimes I do feel sad. There are times that I get emotional—especially when I talk to myself in the mirror. I think I told you way back that my psychiatrist suggested that exercise. It really works for me. I talk to myself now about forgiveness and love. I have forgiven myself for the times I wasn't so nice to Flora during our marriage. When Flora was still alive, while stroking her arm or hair I would tell her how sorry I was about my behavior in the past. This felt like a cleansing and changed our relationship. Being a caregiver has changed me so much. I went from being someone who was impatient and stubborn to a loving and accepting man. As I think about it, I'm grateful that I was able to care for Flora so many years.
>
> I think, too, that one thing that helped me in my grieving is the fact that I joined a bereavement group. We are going through the grieving process step-by-step. Just as it was empowering to be in the caregiver support group, so is it

with the bereavement group. I don't feel isolated. I hear others who feel and think as I do, and we sympathize, inspire, and encourage each other.

So you know, I've been in a relationship with a wonderful woman for five years now. She is nonjudgmental and has keen insight into all sorts of issues. In all this time we've never had any negative words. My family is very accepting of her. What's most amazing to me is that I could love two women at the same time. Having a caring companion with whom I could talk, share dinners, or go to the movies really helped me feel less lonely.

My kids have told me that I was a caring and loving caregiver. They are grateful and very pleased with the job I did in caring for Flora. Other caregivers at the nursing home have told me the same thing. I remember what Carolyn said in group the day I came in to tell everyone that Flora had died. She said that no one could have been so dedicated for the length of time that I had been. She was quite impressed with my skills as a caregiver. I think I have been very fortunate. I look at my life, and I reckon I have had a darn good one.

Nate is 100 percent correct here. He is now eighty-three years old—a young eighty-three in that he definitely doesn't feel his age. He worked until he was seventy-five. Physically, he is very fit, and although he's had hip replacement surgery, he's very active. He swims for an hour every day and then exercises for an additional hour. His attitude continues to be very positive, and he feels he has a lot to look forward to. At the time that we spoke, he was planning what sounded like a wonderful cruise to the Caribbean—a return to some of the islands that he and Flora had visited years ago when he was in the service.

Here's to Nate! Hip hip hooray! Keep on enjoying life!

As Jack Kornfield says in the book *A Grateful Heart*, "At the end of life our questions are very simple: Did I live a full life? Did I love well?"

GETTING STARTED

Eugenia

Eugenia's striving to find renewed meaning in her life gives us cause for celebration of the human spirit. Like so many caregivers, her very active social life had disintegrated as she had devoted more and more time to caring for Jack. Over time, one by one, she had dropped commitments that had given her a great deal of satisfaction and fulfillment. Jack had been dead for four months now. Eugenia was feeling unsettled and lonely and felt that her life no longer had purpose.

> The other day as I sat at the breakfast table finishing my coffee, I thought, "What am I going to do today? What am I going to do with the rest of my life?" It was frightening to have no order, no plan. I was feeling so discombobulated, plus I was lonely. I'd had to turn friends down so often while caring for Jack, that the phone had stopped ringing a long time ago. As you know, I'd also withdrawn from the lawn bowling team that I played on for ten years. They called occasionally to see how I was doing or to encourage me to come back and play, but eventually they gave up on me, too. Once Jack became so agitated I even stopped going to church.
>
> So there I sat. Hoping the phone would ring but knowing it wouldn't. Suddenly, the lightbulb went on in my head. I realized I would live in utter loneliness if I didn't take the bull by the horns. Enough! I picked up the phone, called my friend Aida, and asked her if she could go to lunch sometime. She was surprised and seemed really happy to hear from me. She mentioned that Marge would surely want to join us but wondered if she would since her macular degeneration had gotten so bad that she was no longer able to drive. I was shocked to hear this. Had I really been so out of touch as to

> not know that this had happened to Marge? She had been so independent; I knew coping with this handicap was probably very difficult for her. She lived in my neighborhood, so I offered to pick her up. We three had our lunch date and had a great time. In catching up, however, Marge told us how frustrating daily chores were for her now that she had lost so much of her vision. She was particularly irked that she had to pay drivers or hire teenagers to run errands for her. I offered to be her driver once or twice a week, as I had to run my own errands anyway. Besides, she was great company, and we could make an outing of it and then have dinner together. This turned out to be of significant benefit to both of us. Being alone for the evening meal is still one of the hardest things for me to get used to.
>
> The lawn bowling is another exciting story. Quite coincidentally, around this same time, I ran into Pete from my old lawn bowling team, at the drugstore. He said they'd be starting a new season in September and could really use another player. My knees had grown so stiff since I stopped doing my exercises. However, I told Pete that if I could get these old bones and muscles back in shape in the next two months, I just might join in again. With a little serendipity and a lot of my own initiative, I plan to get back into the swing of things again.

You can expect that living alone will, at times, be challenging and some days more difficult than others. Picking up the phone to make that first call is the hardest. Remember that the resistance you feel is more de-energizing than actually making the call. You may need to give yourself a real talking to and tell yourself that no one is going to do it for you. Whether taking this step opens one door to reclaiming aspects of your life that were important to you before you started caregiving, or gives you the impetus to make a second or third call, the important thing is to just do it. You are well rehearsed by now with being creative and taking command. After all, you have had to be in charge of providing care for your spouse, taking the initiative, and constantly doing battle with the effects of Alzheimer's. Whether you realize it or not, you've been very effective, too. Now is the time to value and honor your life and, by so doing, embrace the challenge of confronting the inherent loneliness and isolation that may have become pervasive during your caregiving years. Frankl refers to this as "the existential vacuum—a feeling of emptiness and meaninglessness."

Think about what has been, is, or could be meaningful to you at this time in your life. What can you live for? What dreams or fantasies capture your imagination? What desires fill you with hope and passion? The answers to these questions do not have to be complicated or extraordinary. They are usually grounded in common sense and are realistically attainable.

You may find it helpful to think about easing back into old, or starting new, activities or relationships slowly, one at a time. First choose an action or activity that is the least risky or intimidating, like Eugenia did in calling an old friend. Start there and then slowly introduce more pleasurable and fulfilling pursuits. Even the most rudimentary activities can bring vitality and vibrancy to your life. To repeat the concept we discussed earlier in this book: Our drive for a sense of belonging, the raison d'etre, the link with significant others in our life, never fades. We feel happier and healthier when we are involved in meaningful relationships with others and have a social network and support system. The older we get, the more satisfaction we enjoy in just being ourselves and feeling a sense of mastery over our lives.

This is a time for you to consciously and actively choose to be more optimistic and sanguine. As Martin Seligman says in his book *Learned Optimism,* "Optimism is a tool to help the individual achieve the goals that he has set for himself. It is in the choice of the goals themselves that meaning—or emptiness—resides." He continues, "Optimism is good for us. It is also more fun: What goes on in our head from minute to minute is more pleasant."

SUCCESSFULLY COMING FULL CIRCLE

As we have come full circle—from the taking on of the caregiver role, to where that challenge has been triumphantly accomplished and life is re-created—we'd like to reflect on examples of optimism. Stan's story will tell it all. One could marvel at his optimism throughout his wife, Lucille's, illness. His positive attitude and his self-confidence were apparent in the way he has always lived his life.

Stan

Stan was a large hulk of a man, a retired Navy officer, who'd come up through the ranks, surviving World War II as a gunner's mate. He had, in the course of our visits, related many of his war stories. He and Lucille lived very modestly in the same house that they bought before his retirement from the Navy, where they had also raised a son, their only child. He took great pride in the remodeling he had done over the years, particularly the addition of a kitchenette. After being retired for a short while, he became antsy and took a part-time job as maintenance man at his church. The added income seemed less important than Stan's feeling that he was doing something worthwhile, and he enjoyed socializing with the minister, church ladies, and parishioners.

Once he had become a caregiver, he had also allied himself with the senior center, attending the caregivers' group and eventually utilizing their day care for Lucille. He initiated monthly spaghetti suppers in his home for the workers at the center, to show his gratitude for their hard work. Toward the end of Lucille's battle with Alzheimer's, he arranged for aides to come in and help with her care. Since he could still lift her quite easily, he and the aide would work together in attending to Lucille's activities of daily living.

Their son, busy with his own career, was not actively involved in caring for Lucille but gave Stan enormous support by coming over several evenings during the week just to visit. Thus, Stan was never isolated. Shortly after Lucille died, I came over for our biannual interview. As I approached the door, I could smell spaghetti sauce cooking.

> Well, Mary, things are sure quiet around here these days; in fact, too quiet, so I decided to do something about it. But let me tell you about my Lucille first. I guess I was really blessed to have had such a wonderful marriage. Yep! When I look back, I was real lucky. Lucille was a Navy nurse, you know. That's how we met. I used to tease her that I married her because I knew she could take care of me in my old age. When Lucille got Alzheimer's, it hit me like a ton of bricks. I couldn't believe it could be happening to her—to us. I thought Alzheimer's would kill the both of us. And sometimes, looking at the hard times, I thought it might kill me before it got Lucille. Every day, every day, the stress of it didn't let up. But I'm stubborn, and I decided I was going to deal with this thing and take care of Lucille to the end.
>
> I would often think that it was trouble to be so in love, especially when I would put her to bed and we'd say our prayers and I'd ask "Why?" But each day I made it through—not on my own you know. It took a whole crew. I may be proud but I ain't stupid. I knew when I was in over my head. There are a lot of good people out there who are willing to help if you just ask. I'm talking about all the folks at the senior center in the support group and in day care and I can't forget how great my boy was in helping keep the ship steady and afloat. Well, Lucille's gone now. I've never cried so hard. I think about her every day, especially all the good times. But I have plenty still to do before the good Lord takes me. I had begun to refinish the pews at church but got behind when Lucille worsened, and you know there's

always more fixin' to do in that old building. Some of the church gals have been bringing the casseroles and now started inviting me over. I'm thinking on that. My son is saying maybe we should move in together. I'm thinking on that, too. I'm having all the helpers from the senior center over for spaghetti tonight. It's been too long since we've had a little repast together at my house.

In the six years that I had known Stan, his caregiving role in reality was not any easier than anyone else's. Alzheimer's does not discriminate. However, in carrying out his role, his "orders," as he would say, he was truly successful. What does make the difference? Let's compile a list using Stan as an example:

1. He loved his wife deeply and they had a good marriage.

2. He was able to separate the person, Lucille, from the disease.

3. Stan came into his role of caregiving with a positive sense of self-esteem and adaptive skills (action versus reaction).

4. He never lost a sense of optimism, which helped him rally against feelings of hopelessness.

5. He knew his own limits and was willing to reach out for help.

6. Whether an evening visit from his son, attending a support group, or working at the church, he did not isolate himself. He maintained a social life and nurtured his altruism.

7. Stan had a sense of humor and also a candor. He was willing to express his feelings but knew not to judge them or beat himself up over them.

AND YOU SHALL TRIUMPH

With a little faith, hope, and optimism you will prevail. Each of you brings into your role of caregiver a long history of achievements, knowledge, skills, and personality traits that will serve as the essence of your success. Inner wisdom and strength accrued over time often lie dormant or go unrecognized until you are faced with adversity. In confronting the challenges of caregiving, you will learn to mobilize that wisdom and strength—that power within you—and rise above your perceived limitations in order to adapt and cope effectively. Would we ever have believed that Leonard would be curling Rene's hair or Thelma would enjoy investing in the stock market?

Don't allow negative feelings to get the better of you. As anger, frustration, and guilt intensify, stop to look them in the eye, name them, and remind yourself that it is normal to have these emotions. By acknowledging them in this way, you will learn to move beyond their debilitating effects and proceed more calmly and clearly in seeking a solution to the provocative situation. Remember that it is your thoughts and beliefs that influence your feelings, and that your thoughts, reactions, and behavior can be changed for the better. You will be able to take events in your stride—one adaptive step at a time.

Learn all that you can about Alzheimer's disease so that you can gain control and competency in caring for your loved one. This will alleviate many fears of the unknown and dispel any myths about the disease that could impair your ability to deal with it.

Open your treasure chest of friends and family who are readily willing to provide practical help for you and your spouse as well as encouragement, love, and emotional support in this time of transitory stress and fragility. Strive to maintain your relationships and outside activities so that isolation does not hold you hostage to this illness.

Join a support group led by an experienced and competent facilitator. Inevitably, you will find that you'll be a stranger only for a very short time. It is here that you will be welcomed with open hearts and open arms and come to experience a true sense of belonging. The commonality of being with other unique individuals who are also caring for an Alzheimer's loved one creates a phenomenal healing bond.

Humbly accept that you are not invincible. Acknowledge your human frailties with compassion and acceptance. You are a worthy opponent of Alzheimer's disease. It cannot overpower you unless you allow it to. Know when to retreat, when to rearm, when to restrategize, and when to call in the troops for fortification.

There are no magical solutions for adjusting to the countless losses and the unremitting cycle of transitions that occur in Alzheimer's disease. Many of you have told us that being a caregiver is the hardest job you've ever taken on. But we have witnessed your strength, creativity, resiliency, and tenacity, which have allowed you to cope successfully with Alzheimer's disease and emerge transformed, fully cognizant of your infinite wholeness.

To "our" caregivers: It is you who have been the triumphant heroes and heroines of *Staying Connected While Letting Go: The Paradox of Alzheimer's Caregiving*. If by retelling your stories we have helped others to come to terms with Alzheimer's, to attain clarity and reason around negative emotions, to assume a greater level of optimism and competency, and, paradoxically and finally, to stay together with their loved one while letting go, then we can end this book knowing that we have achieved what we set out to do. Our grateful hearts and best wishes extend to all of you.

BIBLIOGRAPHY

1. Alterra, Aaron. (2000). *The Caregiver: A Life with Alzheimer's*. Sourth Royalton, VT: Steerforth Press.
2. American Psychiatric Association. (1994). *Diagnostic and Statistical Manual of Mental Disorders*, 4th ed. Washington, D.C.: American Psychiatric Association.
3. Beck, Aaron T. (1979). *Cognitive Therapy and the Emotional Disorders*. New York: Meridian.
4. Chodron, Pema. (2001). *The Places That Scare You*. Boston: Shambhala.
5. Cousins, Norman. (1979). *Anatomy of an Illness*. New York: W. W. Norton and Company.
6. Deane, Barbara. (1989). *Caring for Your Aging Parents*. Colorado Springs: Navpress.
7. Dreikurs, Rudolf. (1967). *Psychodynamics, Psychotherapy, and Counseling*. Chicago: Alfred Adler Institute of Chicago.
8. Frankl, Viktor E. (1959, first translation). *Man's Search for Meaning*. Boston: Beacon Press Books.
9. Genevay, Bonnie. May 1997. "Help Older Adults Overcome 'Intimacy Void.' " *Parent Care Advisor* (May 1997).

10. Gleick, James. (1998). *Chaos: Making a New Science*, New York: Penguin Books.
11. Gruetzner, Howard. (1988). *Alzheimer's: A Caregiver's Guide and Sourcebook.* New York: John Wiley & Sons, Inc.
12. Haisman, Pam. (1998). *Alzheimer's Disease: Caregivers Speak Out.* Fort Myers, FL: Chippendale House Publishers.
13. Kornfield, Jack. (1994). *A Grateful Heart.* Berkeley, CA: Conari Press.
14. Lustbader, Wendy, and Hooyman, Nancy R. (1986). *Taking Care of Aging Family Members—A Practical Guide.* New York: The Free Press.
15. Mace, Nancy L., and Rabins, Peter V. (1981). *The 36-Hour Day.* Baltimore: Johns Hopkins University Press.
16. Nuland, Sherwin B. (1994). *How We Die.* New York: Alfred A. Knopf, Inc.
17. Powell, Lenore S., and Courtice, Katie. (1983). *Alzheimer's Disease: A Guide for Families.* Reading, MA: Addison-Wesley Publishing Company.
18. Rando, Therese A., ed. (2000). *Clinical Dimensions of Anticipatory Mourning.* Champaign, IL: Research Press.
19. Seligman, Martin E. P. (1991). *Learned Optimism.* New York: A. A. Knopf.

ABOUT THE AUTHORS

Sandy Braff

Sandy Braff was born in Johannesburg, South Africa, and came to the USA in 1967. She has been a licensed marriage and family therapist (MFT), since 1984. She is in private practice in San Diego, California. She has dedicated her career to educating and counseling caregivers and family members of Alzheimer's patients, guiding them to successfully adapt to the profound stressors of dealing with Alzheimer's disease. Since 1989 she has voluntarily facilitated a weekly Alzheimer's Caregiver's Support Group for the San Diego Alzheimer's Association. Sandy is also on the Speaker's Bureau of the local association and has presented to many organizations on various topics related to Alzheimer's disease and caregiving issues.

Mary Rose Olenik

As a staff research associate in the Department of Psychiatry at the University of California, San Diego, Mary Rose Olenik conducted over 300 interviews every six months with Alzheimer's caregivers. Although the research study focused on stress as it affects immunity in the spousal caregiver, Mary Rose was profoundly impressed with the caregivers' stories of courage, compassion, adaptation, and the paradox of staying connected while letting go, which were consequential to the data. Ms. Olenik recently moved to New Hampshire, where she plans to continue her work with caregivers and senior advocacy.

INDEX

Abraham
and placement, 183
acceptance, 151
activities of daily living (ADL), 77, 159
Adele
and placement, 178
adult living facilities, 183
advanced directives, 214. *See also* extraordinary measures; living wills
aggression, 98
agitated behaviors, 78
Al
and sexual intimacy, 129
Alterra, Aaron, 66, 245
Alzheimer's Associations
and legal issues, 29
and support groups, 43
and support resources, 22
Alzheimer's Caregiver Research Study, 3, 128
Alzheimer's Disease: A Guide for Families, 246
Alzheimer's Disease: Caregivers Speak Out, 246
Alzheimer's: A Caregiver's Guide and Sourcebook, 246
American Psychiatric Association, 245
Anatomy of an Illness, 111, 245
Andy
and placement, 169
Angela
and compassion, 151
and death, 217
and disclosure, 40
and extramarital relationships, 192
and first encounters, 11
and guilt, 93
and health issues, 101
and placement, 172, 176
and sexual intimacy, 128
anger, 24, 150, 159, 177
Anka
and resentment, 88
antidepressants, 12, 98, 233
antipsychotics, 98
arguments, 12, 51
attention, 76
attorneys, 103
avoidance, 63

Beck, Aaron T., 245
Bella
and humor, 114
bereavement support, 233, 235

INDEX

Bernice
  and resentment, 90
Betty
  and isolation, 62
  and placement, 181
Bill
  and changing roles, 117
  and companions, 140
  and diagnosis, 21
  and difficult behaviors, 80
  and extramarital relationships, 194
  and home care, 145
  and isolation, 62
  and material possessions, 228
  and placement, 180
Bob
  and day care, 138
boundaries, 32
brain autopsies, 220, 224
brain deterioration, 15, 19, 49
brain tumors, 19
breaks, 88, 95, 105, 135, 166
Bud
  and death, 224
  and diagnosis, 23
  and late middle stage, 157
burnout, 159, 166, 173
butterfly effect, 14

care facilities, 179
Caregiver: A Life with Alzheimer's, 66, 245
caregivers
  as whole people, 32
  emotional effects on, 1
  health issues of, 42
Caring for Your Aging Parents, 245
Carolyn
  and acceptance, 151
  and communication, 50
  and day care, 143
  and difficult behaviors, 80
  and extramarital relationships, 192
  and frustration, 107
  and material possessions, 228
catastrophic reaction, 50
catching up, 238
Chaos Theory, 14
Chaos: Making a New Science, 245
children, 39, 165
Chodron, Pema, 232, 245
Clinical Dimensions of Anticipatory Mourning, 214, 246
closure, 200, 220, 224, 235
cognitive function, 19
Cognitive Therapy and the Emotional Disorders, 245
cognitive therapy approach, 2, 75
coma, 205, 212
commitments, 195
communication, 24, 159, 164, 205
community resources, 164
compassion, 151
concentration, 76
confusion, 76
control, 38, 172, 175, 210
conversations, 45, 49
coordination, 159
Cosby, Bill, 114
Courtice, Katie, 246
Cousins, Norma, 111, 245
cures, 85

Darlene
  and placement, 185
day care, 94, 137, 164
Deane, Barbara, 245
decisions, 60, 96, 158
defense mechanisms, 81, 85
dehydration, 211
delusions, 78
Dementia of the Alzheimer's Type (DAT), 19
denial, 34, 41, 59
Denise
  and role changes, 34
dependence, 205
depression, 12, 19
despair, 74
diagnoses, 13
Diagnostic and Statistical Manual of Mental Disorders, 245
Dick
  and fear, 97
dignity, 54
Dreikurs, Rudolf, 58, 93, 245
drug trials, 19
dry mouth, 212
Durable Powers of Attorney, 28

early years, 12. *See* first encounters
eating, 205, 211
edema, 212
Edith
  and denial, 59
education, 63, 75, 86, 94
Edward
  and denial, 59
Eli
  and resentment, 90

Elizabeth
and denial, 83
and fear, 99
and isolation, 152
and placement, 173
Ellen
and first encounters, 15
Elliott
and placement, 62, 181
Elsie
and home care, 145
emergency plans, 102
emotional bonds, 8
emotional reactions, 50
Ernie
and placement, 185
Estelle
and placement, 179
ethics of disclosure, 22
Eugenia
and moving on, 237
Evelyn
and guilt, 93
extramarital relationships, 193
extraordinary measures, 218. *See also* advanced directives

facial expressions, 76
faith, 151
family disease, 167
family meetings, 41, 174
Fay
and humor, 113
feelings, negative, 54
fetal positions, 205
finances, 96, 103, 119, 146, 169
first encounters, 8, 11
Flora
and changing roles, 117
and day care, 139
and death, 221
and difficult behaviors, 81
and final stages, 202
and frustration, 108
and health issues, 102
and placement, 190
and sexual intimacy, 55
fluid retention, 212
Foley catheters, 212
fondling, 127
forgetfulness, 14
Frank
and changing roles, 121
and denial, 84
Frankl, Viktor E., 231, 245
Fred
and home care, 145
friendships, 28, 61
Fritz
and resentment, 88
frustration, 13, 159, 177
full-time nursing, 171

genetic implications, 221
Genevay, Bonnie, 125, 245
Gerhard
and health issues, 100
Gilbert
and advanced directives, 170, 207
Gleick, James, 14, 245
government agencies, 164
Grant, Igor, 3
Grateful Heart, 236, 246
Gray
and changing roles, 119
grief, 175, 200
Gruetzner, Howard, 246
guilt, 87, 129, 132, 172
Gus
and respite, 148

Haisman, Pam, 246
Hal
and placement, 179
hallucinations, 78
Haloperidol, 99
Hannah
and sexual behavior, 56
Harry
and humor, 113
Harvey
and denial, 83
and fear, 99
and placement, 173
Hazel
and changing roles, 118
and companions, 140
and diagnosis, 21
and difficult behaviors, 80
and home care, 146
and isolation, 62
and placement, 180
health care services, 136
health problems
of caregivers, 100, 137
Hedda
and placement, 183
Helga
and participatory grief, 213

Help Older Adults Overcome Intimacy Void, 245
helplessness, 74
Herb
and respite, 147
home care, 144, 160, 164
Hooyman, Nancy R., 246
hospice, 214, 221
hospice care, 169
How We Die, 246
Hugh
and first encounters, 15
humor, 28, 107, 152
hypertension, xvii

Imelda
and material possessions, 229
impatience, 13
in-home care, 137
incontinence, 142, 159
inner voices, 37
intervention, 173
intolerance, 13
isolation, 79, 123, 152, 170, 236

Jan
and day care, 138
Jane
and arguments, 51, 150
and children's involvement, 165
and day care, 141
and disclosure, 25
and first encounters, 7
and isolation, 60, 64
and material possessions, 228
and mutuality, 47
and sexual intimacy, 112
Jean
and respite, 148
Jenny
and extramarital relationships, 132
Joan
and difficult behaviors, 81
and disclosure, 27
Joe
and death, 217
and disclosure, 41
and first encounters, 11
and health issues, 101
and placement, 172, 176
and sexual intimacy, 128
John
and communication, 50
and day care, 143
and difficult behaviors, 80
and frustration, 107
Joy
and respite, 147
judgments, 17

Kornfield, Jack, 236, 246

Lars
and participatory grief, 213
Learned Optimism, 239, 246
legal conservatorships, 29
legal documents, 103
Leonard
and changing roles, 122
and day care, 143
and extramarital relationships, 192
and patience, 150
and sexual intimacy, 130
life-sustaining treatments, 210
Lily
and fear, 97
living wills, 28, 103. *See also* advanced directives
loneliness, 65, 126, 131
lucidity, 34
Lustbader, Wendy, 246

Mac
and arguments, 51, 150
and children's involvement, 165
and day care, 141
and disclosure, 25
and isolation, 60, 64
and sexual intimacy, 112
Mace, Nancy L., 246
magnetic resonance imaging (MRI), 19
Mamie
and death, 224
and diagnosis, 23
and late middle stage, 157
Man's Search for Meaning, 231, 245
Mannie
and caregiver reactions, 53
and extramarital relationships, 192
and family meetings, 41
and guilt, 94
and humor, 151
and material possessions, 228
and moving on, 232
and placement, 171
and sexual intimacy, 129
and tentative diagnosis, 18
Martha
and placement, 169

masturbation, 127, 129
material possessions, 227, 230
Max
  and sexual behavior, 56
May
  and first encounters, 12
medications, 19, 99, 212
memorial services, 235
memory, 14, 18, 19, 76, 158
morphine, 212
motor skills, 76
mourning, 214
moving on, 233
muscle jerks, 76

naso-gastric suction tubes, 212
Nate
  and changing roles, 117
  and day care, 139
  and death, 221
  and difficult behaviors, 81
  and extramarital relationships, 132, 191
  and final stages, 202
  and frustration, 108
  and health issues, 102
  and moving on, 235
  and placement, 172, 190
  and sexual intimacy, 55
National Institutes of Health (NIH), 3
Ned
  and respite, 147
negative feelings, 79, 87, 111
negative thoughts, 92
Neil
  and role changes, 34
neurofibrillary tangles, 221
neurologists, 13, 19
neuropsychologists, 19
Nuland, Sherwin B., 246
nurturers, 116

obligations, 95
Ogden
  and placement, 178
Olga
  and respite, 148
Olivia
  and health issues, 100
Olympia
  and changing roles, 121
  and denial, 84
opiate derivatives, 212
optimism, 37
orgasm, 129

pain medications, 212
palliative care, 211
paranoia, 97
Parkinson's disease, 19
patience, 150
Patterson, Thomas L., 3
Paul
  and first encounters, 7
  and mutuality, 46
Peg
  and sexual intimacy, 129
personal belongings. *See* material possessions
personality changes, 15, 18, 76
pessimism, 34
Phil
  and anger, 71
  and difficult behaviors, 80
  and disclosure, 40
  and first encounters, 17
  and frustration, 106
  and sexual intimacy, 55
Phyllis
  and placement, 170
physical examinations, 19
physical intimacy, 125
Places That Scare You, 232, 245
playfulness, 114
Powell, Lenore S., 246
presence, 66
protectors, 116
psychiatrists, 20
Psychodynamics, Psychotherapy, and Counseling, 58, 245

Rabins, Peter V., 246
Rachel
  and caregiver reactions, 53
  and guilt, 94
  and sexual intimacy, 130
  and tentative diagnosis, 18
Rando, Therese, 214
Rando, Therese A., 246
reasoning, 17
rejection, 63
relationships
  and education, 64
  and late middle stage, 160
  changes in, 45
  impact on, 14
  protecting, 31
  reestablishing, 239
relatives, 61
release, 23, 200, 219, 235

Rene
  and changing roles, 122
  and day care, 143
  and patience, 150
  and sexual intimacy, 130
repetitive behaviors, 78
research, 19
resentment, 159, 173, 177
respite, 88, 95, 105, 135, 144, 166
restlessness, 76
retirement facilities, 101, 179
Richard
  and changing roles, 120
  and day care, 140, 142
  and difficult behaviors, 80
  and final stages, 199
  and first encounters, 16
  and personality changes, 48
  and role changes, 33
Rosa
  and advanced directives, 207

safety, 26, 35
San Diego Alzheimer's Association, 2
self-loathing, 94
self-respect, preserving, 23
Seligman, Martin E. P., 37, 239, 246
senescence, 63
senile plaques, 221
separation, 175
sexual intimacy, 54, 66, 125, 189
shadowing, 159
shared delusions, 52
short term care, 101
sleep patterns, 78
societal boundaries, 16
Sol
  and humor, 114
Sophie
  and role changes, 35
spouses. *See* caregivers
Stan
  and guilt, 93
  moving on, 240
Stella
  and children's involvement, 166
Steve
  and difficult behaviors, 81
stress, 36, 153, 164
strokes, 19, 49
sundowning, 76
  and anger, 48, 72
  and belonging, 65
  and communication, 52
  and family involvement, 164
  and gender differences, 116, 122
  and new communities, 26
  and placement, 173
  and problem behaviors, 98
  and resentment, 89
Sylvia
  and anger, 71
  and difficult behaviors, 80
  and disclosure, 40
  and first encounters, 17
  and frustration, 106
  and material possessions, 229
  and sexual intimacy, 55
sympathy, 62
symptoms, 14

Taking Care of Aging Family Members—A Practical Guide, 246
Thelma
  and changing roles, 118
therapists, 98, 103, 105, 137
36-Hour Day, 246
three-tier facilities, 178
Tom
  and disclosure, 27
Tony
  and role changes, 35
transient ischemic attacks (TIAs), 49
turmoil, 12, 31
twitching, 76

verbal abuse, 97
Veronica
  and denial, 82
violence, 96
vitamin deficiencies, 19

Winston
  and first encounters, 12
working, 186

Yvette
  and changing roles, 120
  and day care, 140, 142
  and difficult behaviors, 80
  and extramarital relationships, 194
  and final stages, 199
  and first encounters, 16
  and personality changes, 48
  and role changes, 33

Zeke
  and denial, 82